WIN/WIN OUTCOMES:

A PHYSICIAN'S NEGOTIATING GUIDE

SEYMOUR J. BURROWS

Pluribus Press Inc.
DIVISION OF TEACH 'EM INC

Library of Congress Catalog Card Number:
84-60125

International Standard Book Number:
0-931028-46-9

Pluribus Press, Inc., Division of Teach'em, Inc.
160 East Illinois Street
Chicago, Illinois 60611

Printed in the United States of America

To

James H. Sammons M.D., who, as Executive Vice-President of the American Medical Association, foresaw the need for physicians to understand and practice the art of negotiation and established the AMA's Department of Negotiation in 1975; Ike Mayeda and Jerry Clousson, who joined with me in making Dr. Sammons's dream come alive; and Louise, my patient and understanding spouse, who put up with my messy work habits.

Contents

INTRODUCTION

Truth is a constant variable. We seek it, we find it, our viewpoint changes—and the truth changes to meet it.

William J. Mayo, M.D.

Physicians often are great and wonderful people. But many are grievously naive when confronted with sharp business practices. Confident in their ability to cure or alleviate illness, pain and suffering, they assume that the respect and appreciation they are accorded for their medical skills will motivate those for whom and with whom they work. While at one time this may have been true, in today's litigious climate it is no longer the case. This is clearly seen in media and other attacks now routinely made against physicians by government regulators, hospital administrations, public interest groups, and unhappy patients and their attorneys.

Six years of working with physicians under the auspices of the American Medical Association have convinced me that too many of them do not know how to negotiate. Physicians should not come to a bargaining table less well prepared than those whom they meet there. Negotiation involves more than saying what you want or expect to get, and having it handed to you without opposition. The days of easy acquiescence and blank checks have ended and the time for negotiation has arrived. The ability to negotiate is a necessary skill for hospital staffs, independent physicians and employed doctors. It can be an extremely useful skill for the medical practitioner as well.

Learning to negotiate in adversary situations can add flexibility and resourcefulness to other relationships, both business and social. The principles and techniques through which the negotiation process works can be applied to an unlimited number of circumstances.

What is there for physicians to negotiate? Why should doctors have to negotiate?

Every day, in innumerable ways and situations, physicians are faced with problems and conditions that require conscious or unconscious involvement with the process. Most of the time they do not realize that they are negotiating. Because communications are not being exchanged in a formal negotiating atmosphere, or situation, much negotiation is not recognized for what it is. But, convincing a patient of what may be best for him, promoting an idea to one's peers or associates, or expressing or clarifying one's position is, essentially, negotiation.

Because most of their negotiating experiences have produced less than satisfactory results, physicians' negative negotiating attitudes can be ascribed to largely unstructured or unconscious resentment at having to maneuver in an unfamiliar discipline. What I will try to do in this book is establish a format for developing a process of negotiating with which you can feel comfortable, and direct your thoughts and actions toward improving your negotiating skills.

However, as physicians well know, a text can only illustrate suggestive approaches to a problem. You can learn new and better ways to organize your thoughts by reading, but the only way to improve your results is by observation and practice. As I will often repeat in the following pages, you can become a better negotiator—as long as you do it in the manner that is most comfortable to you—within the framework of the process that will be described.

1
THE NEED FOR NEGOTIATIONS

Dimidium facti qui caepit habet (He who has begun has the work half done)

Horace

Let us begin with the obvious question: What are some of the areas in which physicians are, will be, or may be, negotiating?

For physicians:

Medical staff bylaws, rules and regulations;

Due process;

Utilization reviews, both as reviewer and reviewee and now application of DRGs;

Staff privileges;

Office management;

Patients and their insurors.

For independent contractors:

Contracts and other forms of agreement and their enforcement;

Intrastaff relationships;

Interstaff relationships;

Employee supervision;

Partners and/or other practitioners of the same specialty;

Third parties (insurors, regulators, etc.).

For medical staffs and their governing bodies:

Quality care issues;

Application of DRGs and other regulatory infringements;

Fees for hospital-based physicians and exclusive contracts;

Closed or open staffs and privilege deliniation;

Hill-Burton fulfillments to treat indigent and Medicaid patients;

Expansion of nurses' duties into traditional areas of medical competence and patient care;

Ditto expansionist attempts of other paramedical and technician groups;

Privileges for licensed non-physician professionals such as podiatrists, dentists, and chiropacters, and non-scientific healers who, in some states may be licensed on a limited basis;

Laboratory procedures requested by chiropracters and others;

Patient grievances and the hospital's handling thereof;

Public relations.

For medical societies and their representatives:

Representing the profession locally, vis-a-vis hospitals and their associations;

Intragroup relationships for dispute settlements;

Disciplinary and ombudsman situations;

Representing members in public and semi-public situations;

Protection of medical privilege and status; etc., and in

Governmental and insuror situations such as: State welfare departments:

Procedural codes and payments;

Turnaround times for bill submission and payment;

Fee schedules and fee reviews;

Advertising codes and review;

Grievance machinery and usage;

Screened data for disciplinary action, other types of review;

Payments for, and definition of, "new" and improved procedures;

Release of payment and other information to the media and the public;

Updating of requirements and interpretations that may be imposed by a copaying agency;

Blue Cross/Blue Shield: (both as a major government carrier and private patients' representative)

All of the above and following, plus

Cost containment efforts such as retroactive procedural reviews, prospective payment practices, and elective admission restrictions;

Payments for services not requiring hospital admission;

Free and open communication to avoid dictatorial imposition of planned reductions or restrictions;

Private insurance carriers:

Most of the above, plus

Second opinion programs, their marketing and payment;

Laboratory procedures and fee schedules;

Billing reviews and procedure updating;

Utilization reviews;

Publicity usage without prior notice, medical clearance and discussion;

Advance notice to or through the society of procedural changes in sufficient time to allow discussion.

A current bromide goes "If you are not part of the solution, you must be part of the problem." You cannot sit back, isolating yourself and your practice from what is going on in the socioeconomics of medicine. Such detachment, with the excuse that you are "too busy," or "It has nothing to do with my practice," or "Let the AMA take care of it," is no longer available to you. As financial resources diminish; as utilization of benefits for recipients of Medicare and Medicaid, employer-paid and private insurances increase; as competition among the ever-growing pool of your peers becomes more a fact; as the spreading tentacles of coordinated and corporate hospital management reach for your patients through outpatient centers and ambulatory clinics; as you and your peers are increasingly circumscribed by the rules and controls of government and insurance companies; as all payors inspect your billings more cynically because those who pay the premiums are demanding improved controls and "more bang for the buck"; you, individually and collectively, cannot sit back and wait for the AMA or some other dragon-slayer to take up your banner and bring back the good old days. Before "they" tie you into practice restrictions and legalese, you must learn and know how to be as well-prepared and able as are they.

As you read this, make up your mind that "negotiation" and "compromise" are not dirty words. By engaging in the process, you do not in any way denigrate yourself or your professionalism. Make no mistake. Physicians can become successful negotiators—for themselves, for groups they have chosen to represent, and for their publics.

Physicians as Negotiators

What has caused, or created, this need for physicians to become negotiators? Perhaps a quote from an advocate for the other side—an administrator of a teaching hospital—crystallizes the issue:

> Why does a simple undertaking like a physician contract pose any serious difficulties? After all, physicians and hospital leaders are *reasonable* people, working together for a common goal—improved health care for *their* patients. And it is hard to imagine that even the most complex working relationships could not be reduced, somehow, to some fundamental issues that could be incorporated into a working agreement. It is simple in theory, but unfortunately a *Gordian knot* in reality when applied to doctors and hospitals. "*Unknown to the public until only recently is a long-standing feud between hospitals and hospital-based physicians over contractual arrangements and methods of compensation with those specialists*. . . (emphasis author's)[1]

[1]*How To Negotiate Physician Contracts,* Dean F. Grant, p. 2. Second edition 1983. Teach 'em, Inc., Chicago, IL.

Note how the presentation and use of buzz-words immediately puts the physicians in an adversarial position and in the wrong. This chief executive officer (CEO) talks simultaneously of being ''reasonable'' under the threat of a ''Gordian knot'' while being concerned about ''their'' (physicians' *and* hospital leaders') patients. He then puts the negotiating stance into an apparent ''no-win'' frame by characterizing it as a ''long-standing feud.'' Giving the public this slant to the problem tends to make the hospitals the ''good guys'' and put the physicians (with whom we must assume the hospitals want, and need, to work) on the defensive. Our administrator friend goes on to admit that:

> . . . For a whole series of complicated and now regrettable reasons, many hospitals have *allowed* most of their hospital-based specialists to operate with open-ended contracts which at best can be described as lacking common logic and basic economic principles. . .[2]

It is better to put this ''feud'' and the actions that are ''lacking common logic and [ignoring] basic economic principles'' into their proper perspective as a mutual problem, and to give them the open-minded and analytical approach they deserve.

Admittedly, these comments have been presented slightly out of context in order to emphasize that author's use of words. I believe that the origin of these ''open-ended'' contracts rests in the inexperience and lack of training of those who first negotiated them—the administrators and their lawyers whose motivation was not only to increase personal income, but also to minimize apparent employee-type liabilities and benefits, and the physicians who were presented with what appeared to be a ''good thing''. However, the hospital administrators went to school and quickly learned how to use hospital-based physicians' lack of interest and negotiating experience to write contracts that circumscribed the doctors' independence and to use those ''. . . *contractual arrangements and methods of compensation* . . .'' to boost the income from those specialty departments to subsidize other more colorful and costly but unprofitable departments.

Unfortunately, while pushing the income of the subsidizing departments, the hospital administrators used little foresight about the possible negative effects of their ''open-ended'' agreements. When things were going well for hospitals, administrators were content to look the other way. Then, when competition and inflation forced hospitals to respond to financial controls and external agencies, self-protection became an issue. The

[2]ibid: Grant

administrators conveniently forgot or ignored who had instigated these contracts that suddenly were odious. Instead, the administrators joined forces with the regulators and the consumer advocates in decrying the gross incomes of hospital-based and other physicians from whose work their hospitals profited. The onus for "escalating" hospital costs was placed upon the doctors. Now market strictures in health care are forcing the parties to look—together—for publicly and mutually satisfactory solutions. The regulators, the insurors, the employers—as long as they were in good health—wanted an end to escalating costs. (However, when someone requires health care, costs paid by insurance should not be allowed to be a deterrent to getting the best care available.)

To maintain their image and to serve the public consumer advocates, the regulators, the insurors, the employers, and the hospital administrators huddled with their lawyers and their associations and began taking lessons in business practices and negotiating. The physicians, in good faith, continued doing their jobs and, in most cases, paid no attention to the growing tumult. Hospital administrators, encouraged by their education and support staffs, not only began to outnegotiate their "partners" in "working together for a common goal", but also to make up new rules for their working together. Most hospital-based specialists were unaware of the changing climate, along with the rest of the hospital staff.

Targets for Cost-Cutting

Let us look into a little history, since there is obviously no one reason for this attitude reversal on the part of the hospital administrations. The most obvious opponents, if we had to name them, should perhaps be the hospitals and the third-party payors who pass the consumer dollars, or the patients and their insuror representatives. The individual physician as a target for cost-cutting is a less satisfactory target for the general public. As targets and perpetrators of inflated health care costs, the hospitals and the insurors have apparently become allies of a sort, and may have chosen to distract the burden of escalating costs from themselves by putting the blame on the physicians. Why not target those moneybags, the doctors who are in the front line and are readily recognizable? Self preservation has become the goal for the several factions of health care providers. How have we come to these positions?

During World War II, under imposed restrictions, wage increases for workers on the home front were limited, but the unions that supported the president and were vigorously supporting the war effort had to be kept happy and cooperative. The War Labor Board (WLB) discovered a way to work around its own rules. "Fringe benefits." What better way to give Rosie the Riveter and the union leaders something while apparently still staying within their rules? In combination with new Blue Cross/Blue Shield programs that had been established to ensure guaranteed payments for specified hospital and medical services, unions and managements could add to the workers' take-home pay by reducing the occasional cost of medical care, with the blessings of the WLB. The public-spirited leaders of labor, management, and government claimed the credit from the workers and could still claim credit for patriotically holding down wage increases.

Today's profit-metasticizing fringe benefit, health and medical insurance, grew from that limited beginning. The cause for this drain on profits and strain on the costs of doing business, is said not to be the benign negotiation of union and management, but rather the greed of the hospitals and the physicians! Little, if any, credit or recognition is given to the regular expansion of hospital and medical benefits that has been followed by employee utilization. Nor, until recently, has much attention been given to the minimal oversight given to either utilization or payments by employers' or the insurors' claim processing. (The insurors, after all, paid claims as they were authorized by the employers and increased premiums to meet their profit requirements, and the employers expected the insurors to check the bills.)

Then, in 1968, the "Great Society" of President Lyndon Johnson gave us Medicare and Medicaid. As with many political innovations, these grants to the peoples' welfare were implemented with more regard to form and intent than to the substance of utilization and costs. From the beginnings of these plans, bureaucratization was apparently more important than controls or supervision. Utilization zoomed as did the concomitant expense, so that the cost of these programs escalated from the great society payouts in 1967 of 7.4 billion to the 1981 payout of 73.2 billion dollars. Fault had to be found, and the bureaucrats and politicians have made the hospitals and the doctors their scapegoats. Facts such as poor administration, constant expansion of benefits for political advantage and less restricted benefits are cavalierly ignored by those who blame the health care providers.

Cost containment, for some time now, has been the buzz-word for control. The action toward effective cost reduction appears to insist that "something must be done" with pressure, which is placed first on the hospitals. Hospitals, licensed for public benefit, are easy targets, because this is where the largest payouts are made. But the hospitals need help to stay solvent and maintain their services and their staffs. One way to continue to collect the bulk of the public and private monies is to convert "independent contractor" physicians into employees. In this way salaries become part of the total cost of doing hospital business (Part A, Medicare and Medicaid, Blue Cross; etc.). Physician services then are not listed as such, but become an integral part of a functional service cost. Along with these pressures, university programs for hospital administrators—MHA's in the Harvard MBA style—have steadily developed. Hospital administrators by training were encouraged to take more complete control over everything that went on within the hospital.

A number of judicial decisions assessing hospital boards of directors' accountability assisted hospital administrators in their pursuit of administrative control. Darling vs. Charleston Memorial Hospital (1965, Illinois) established the precedent for fundamental responsibility of a hospital for the quality of care within its jurisdiction—medical care by physicians as well as that delivered by the hospitals' non-medical staffs. Two legal theories are the basis for the courts' decisions—*respondeat superior* and corporate responsibility. Under *respondeat superior* the hospital is, or may be assumed to be, the senior in a master/servant relationship, and thus able to control or be responsible for the control of those working within the hospital premises. That control is assumed for both performance of services within the hospital's jurisdiction and for the conduct of those performing those services. This theory, in law, was originally established to cover the employer/employee relationship, but as the courts have become more socially and responsibility cognizant, it has been extended to its current interpretations. The second theory, that of corporate responsibility, asserts that the board of directors and administration of a hospital have ultimate control over the facilities, the rules and procedures for practice.

These theories and their implementation have created a classic *Catch 22* situation for health care professionals. On one hand, the hospitals have been ordered to assume monopolistic control of their facilities with concomitant responsibility for the actions of all who work within that monopoly. On the other hand, this monopolist must maintain a peaceful and ongoing relationship with the physicians who have admitting privileges. The hospital is simultaneously responsible for the conduct of its medical staff while dealing with them as suppliers (or customers, if you will, because the physicians are the prime source of admitted patients). The situation is further skewed by granting, either through subcontracting or assigning restricted services, monopolistic (or exclusive) territorial rights to limited functions within the hospital. Thus, while assuming responsibility for internal control, the hospitals are left open to harrassment by medical specialists who would like to practice as independent members of the hospital medical staff. Relationships are further complicated by government regulations that decree specific amounts of free indigent care while insisting that indigent, Medicare, and Medicaid patients receive care as good as that which private patients receive although the payments will be considerably lower. And, not to be left out of this complicated fiscal fiasco, insurance carriers insist on single-price structures by not permitting differences in charges for procedures performed under different circumstances, such as those services for outpatients and those for inpatients. In effect, while demanding cost-control, the insurors prevent hospitals and their hospital-based medical staffs from competing with other outpatient organizations.

What seems to be developing is a reluctant appreciation of hospital ascendancy in the hospital/physician/patient relationship. Appreciation, not acceptance. While hospital administrations have been given the opportunity to exercise controls that some might label tyrannical, total exploitation is held back by unions of employees and the influence, real or percieved, of professional societies whose cooperation is a necessary adjunct to profitable operation. We are witnessing a classic multi-party negotiating tactic—get the allies to fight among themselves, waste their efforts among themselves, and use their common opponent (insurors, regulators, bureaucrats) to settle issues, to the disadvantage of their allies.

It will do little good for anyone to try to designate a particular culprit for the medical care mess that has developed. The mess is here, now, and should be recognized for what it is. No one participating in health care—patients, physicians, hospitals, insurance carriers, unions, employers, governments with their regulations and bureaucratic functionaries, politicians—is in position to lay blame or claim immunity from fault for cost escalation, overutilization, or proliferation of benefits. The principals in health care, physicians and hospitals, have a common need to work together for their mutual continuation as viable health purveyors, while at the same time working out a means for resolving their differences. For the most part, hospitals have, for some time, been able to protect their interests. Now, physicians, both individually and through their various organizations, will have to be ready and able to stand up and protect themselves when necessary. Negotiation will be the peaceful means available to those who are prepared.

2
WHAT'S IT ALL ABOUT

Don't ever slam a door. You might want to go back.
Don Herold

Negotiation is a problem-solving process. By engaging in the process, two or more parties work to reach a mutually acceptable answer to those matters of concern where they may be in conflict or disagreement. Through the exchange of ideas and information, the parties seek to define the extent of their problems and the alternative solutions available to them. They work to persuade their opponents to modify their goals and expectations as they search for an answer that both parties can live with for the immediate future. Negotiations are ''successful'' when an agreement allows both parties to leave the negotiating arena feeling that they have done their best, and have made the best deal possible *for the present.* Let me emphasize ''for the present'' because that is the essence of negotiating between parties that have an ongoing relationship. Agreements for the future aspects of a continuing relationship are based, in part, on hope as well as upon the past history of the parties. With the passage of time, conditions change and agreements have to be renegotiated. Agreements are good for the parties as long as they are both satisfied by whatever they had set up as a working arrangement. When conditions change, either because of internal needs or external stresses, an updated contractual arrangement must be negotiated.

The Win/Win Outcome

The current buzz-word for a successful settlement is "win/win." The common thread to satisfactory negotiating conclusions is that, in satisfying your own needs with the best current solution you also work to satisfy your opponent's needs in the same manner. As with any draconian solution (i.e., Versailles 1918) where one side gets little or nothing, the ego-need to "get even" will result in troubled administration of the one-sided settlement and more-than-difficult renegotiation. As partners to a negotiated settlement, you and your opponent should have mutual interests. Among these mutual interests are: an interest in maintaining a continuing relationship for your mutual benefit; establishing a clearly defined basis for that continuation; and continuing friendly approaches toward more even-tempered negotiations. The win/win answer to conflict resolution is not being promoted to say that in order to achieve negotiating success one must be prepared to abandon principles. Nor does it recommend such strict adherence to positions that you reach an impasse. Differences of principles and goals often can be utilized to develop flexible alternatives that have a measure of satisfaction for both parties. With each side getting part of what he came to the table for, by each sensibly modifying proposals through cognizance of the opponent's position, both are able to walk away from the table convinced that the current agreement is the best possible for the immediate future. Thus, the results of a successful negotiation are often the outcome of compromise. And, compromise need not be looked upon as inevitable defeat. In fact, most often negotiators, through compromise, work out mutually acceptable solutions that neither party had previously conceived or considered.

Current literature and dramatic lecturers emphasize "how to's" for one-time negotiations—how to overpower your opponent; how to make a better deal at your opponent's expense; how to take advantage of a good-faith opponent; etc. These could be effective if one does not have to meet with that opponent—usually a purchasor or seller—again. But physicians, in most of negotiating situations, should consider the long-term effects of their agreements. While they may take advantage of some of the tactics espoused by the win-at-all-costs advocates, they should do so cautiously, fully aware of the possibilities of revenge if they are too successful. The complexities of actual situations (often difficult to determine or evaluate because of the opponent's mental, attitudinal and organizational background) and the many uncertain realities that negotiators must consider, make any approach other than the win/win framework less than satisfactory for the physician negotiator. By understanding the parameters within which the "other guy" should, or ought to be, operating, you can be practicing in an orderly fashion.

The Win/Lose Failure

One ploy that your opponents might use to effectuate a win-lose settlement is called divide and conquer. Hospital administrators, insurors, politicians, consumer-advocates, media headline-hunters—you name them—will always be ready to invoke this tactic. And quite often, they are successful. It isn't too difficult. Because of physicians' individual independence and the proliferation of specialties and sub-sub-specialty divisions, divide and conquer plays to self-interest. Physicians tend to become over-involved in their areas of specific interest and leave the broader interests of medicine to "George." Thus, primary care physicians, hospital-based physicians, surgeons (a most fertile field for protection of overlapping turfs), employed physicians and physician-supervisors, proliferating paramedical specialists, and technicians who are claiming entrance into what was once sacrosanct medical territory, are all vulnerable to manipulation under the guise of promotion or preservation of self-interest. If you are not prepared to negotiate, individually and collectively, you may well find yourself not only left out, but taken advantage of.

It's important to identify the areas of medicine that are, or may soon be, grounds for negotiating. Pressures are being placed upon the hospital-based physicians who are called independent contractors. If they are still on some form of percentage contract, they are accused of being reimbursed, not for the work they have done, but as a free-ride adjunct to the costs of operation of their department. If they separate-bill for their services, they draw patient complaints because the patients believe that they are being charged twice for the same service. And, if they combine-bill, they run the risk of accounting and/or computer problems with the hospital. Because payment for the services of a hospital-based physician appear more readily acceptable to insurors—and seem to be less-closely audited when buried within the total service charge of the hospital—hospital administrators would prefer having full control of charges under a unified billing. And through the device of "independent contractor" agreements that, when looked at closely, resemble employment contracts in everything but name, it becomes a matter of truly independent survival that hospital-based physicians be ready to negotiate on a near-level with the administrators.

As a practicing physician you may be simon-pure in your practice and the best doctor in the world to your patients. However, that will not stop those numerous and jealous people who are not your patients and who are always ready to point and yell with alarm at their assumption of your greed because their insurance failed to fully cover their bill. At the same time, they do not disapprove—more than likely, they will compliment—the athlete, entertainer or business executive who manipulates a multi-six-figure contract. These complaints over "excessive" charges rarely come down to asking "Why?" After recovering, some patients forget or ignore their insistence under the crisis of illness that they receive "the best that's available, cost is no object." This is an area where it may well be advisable for physicians, and particularly surgeons, to take the initiative to negotiate with their patients.

Strategies and Approaches

Some of the strategies and approaches that will be presented in the following chapters as facets of the negotiation process may not concur with your ideas of interpersonal relations. It is not necessary to put them all to use. It is necessary to be aware of what a less-than-scrupulous opponent may be trying to accomplish at your expense. When you are entering this realm of interpersonal relations called negotiations, you will find a universe very different from the medical world in which you were trained and now work. It is a world of an infinitesimal number of shades of gray, where the absolute blacks and whites become roadblocks to mutually satisfactory agreements.

In any of the situations that have been referred to thus far, and to other situations you may be party to, you will find a need to negotiate. It may be negotiation to maintain certain conditions. As the Red Queen so aptly stated in Lewis Carroll's *Through the Looking Glass,* "Sometimes you have to run as fast as you can just to stay where you are." No one else will do it for you. You may have to engage in what is called retrieval negotiations—situations where something that you gave away in an earlier negotiation or that your opponent appropriated without negotiating now require that you assert your need for change. Or, you may find that you have to engage in developmental negotiations—where new or changed procedures or practices should be recognized by one's opponent. More often than not goals and objectives will fall short of your expectations in a current negotiation. Full appreciation and accomplishment may require a series of negotiations and several agreements over an extended period of time. You are going to have to cultivate patience, tact, and flexibility. As you develop your style, and become comfortable with it, you will achieve more substantive results and will feel better about how you won them.

3
DEFINING TERMS

"The question is," Alice said, "whether you can make words mean so many different things." "The question is," said Humpty Dumpty, "which is to be the master."

Lewis Carroll, Through the Looking Glass

For successful negotiations, it is necessary to discuss the subject in terms both sides can understand. For our mutual understanding of the process, let us define some of those words and terms.

Parties/Opponents/Adversaries

Parties are the people who sit at the negotiating session. They may be *adversaries,* truly out to "get" the other party for whatever reason. We prefer to call the people sitting opposite us *opponents.* An opponent may well be a friend, a person with whom you can openly discuss problems and work out mutually satisfactory solutions and disagreements. Mutual trust and credibility should make up the basic framework that establishes the other negotiator as an opponent rather than an adversary. Negotiations must be looked upon as a playing field, large enough for the parties to go their own way. If they meet head-on, they should have sufficient room to back off a little to work out an accommodation that will permit each to move toward a goal. The longer you are able to prevent that person sitting opposite you from becoming an adversary, the better chance you have of calm and successful negotiations.

Negotiating/Bargaining

Negotiation will be used to embrace the total extent of the relations between the parties. It is intended to include all that takes place, from the moment the parties recognize that they have a mutual problem, to the time that they reach a mutually satisfactory solution and beyond. *Bargaining,* however, will be used in a much narrower sense. When the parties bargain, they are maneuvering for tactical advantage, playing off concessions and counterproposals to come as close to their original goals as they can. While common usage and application have erased much of the distinction between these words to the point that most people use them interchangeably, the difference between the total concept of the process and the more limited give-and-take, or nitty-gritty, of bargaining should be made.

Problems/Disputes/Disagreements

Problems, disagreements and disputes develop in almost any relationship because no elaboration of rules for a working relationship can be established to satisfy the handling of future situations. Problems develop and create disagreements because of structural or human inadequacies in a relationship. Structural inadequacies seem to be built into a relationship because of parties' inability or lack of interest in developing or using some form of adjudication to resolve, if only until another opportunity for negotiation presents itself. Human inadequacies become evident in the form of egos, personal values and other situations where feelings take the place of clear thinking. *Problem-solving,* adjudication by mutual resolution, takes place when either or both parties decide that they cannot continue to live with a situation. Problem-solving as a means of resolving inter- or intraparty disagreements and stresses may be either formal or informal. Such disagreements or disputes should be looked upon as opportunities for mutual solution, and not as intolerable bases for open warfare.

Win/Win, Win/Lose, Lose/Lose, Compromise

Compromise and negotiations should not be looked upon as dirty words. Concessions and compromises may be necessary to maintain a certain relationship or to gain something you desire. A *win/win* situation, mentioned in an earlier chapter, is usually the best solution for negotiators to strive for. Any *win/lose* result will, in time, turn into a *lose/lose* because an opponent who is decisively beaten could decide to retaliate. Compromise, through problem-solving, therefore enables negotiators to work out solutions that help both parties. And, while neither party may be completely satisfied with the compromise result, both can live with it for the immediate future. By thoughtful goal planning, negotiators can avoid what could develop into an ongoing adversarial situation where a mounting lack of trust and credibility eventually has both parties fighting to finishes that help no one.

Demands/Proposals

Demands imply requests at negotiating sessions that the other party is likely to regard as peremptory orders for compliance. *Proposals,* on the other hand, appear as requests for consideration of problems of mutual concern. It is always better to involve the other party in a cooperative effort than to put him in a defensive attitude when negotiating. More on this later.

Bottom Line

Behind the give and take of negotiating lie the minimum results you wish to achieve. As you approach this bottom line, you must stand strong against your opponent.

Strategies/Tactics

Strategies are overall action plans for achieving satisfactory resolution of one's objectives. Strategy development could include establishing ranges for settling your goals; uncovering the limits within which your opponent hopes to settle; identifying the areas of disagreement and potential agreement; establishing a basis for concessions and counteroffers; deciding the attitude or manner that will be used in negotiation; determining how information will be accumulated to support your positions; and preparing for allied support that may be required to pressure your opponent. *Tactics,* on the other hand, are the during-negotiations techniques that help you implement your basic strategies. One caveat must be put forward in connection with any discussion of tactics: don't confuse reasonable tactics with out-and-out game playing or gamesmanship. The use of such game tactics, if played to excess or at the wrong times, will act as a put-down to a competent opponent. Such tactics will be recognized as evidence of bad-faith negotiating or as evidence of someone bargaining from a poorly-supported position, and the same tactics may be used against you.

Power

Negotiating *power* is perceived in many guises. Physicians have a certain amount of built-in power through reputation and status. Those physician services that are recognized as absolute essentials by the opponent may become a basis of power. Negotiating power at times may appear to be one-sided. However, each negotiator has some basis for power, and must determine how to use those bases to his best advantage.

4
BEFORE THE DRAMA: PLANNING AND PREPARATION

In all things, success depends upon previous preparation, and without such preparation there is sure to be no future.

Kung Fu-Tse (Confucius)

Collective bargaining, in the early days of legalized labor-management relations, was characterized as "management bargains while the union collects." In many ways physician negotiations currently appear to be in a similar state, with physicians on the bargaining side. I am reminded of a first negotiation that I chaired for an industrial manufacturer with its union. For about twenty years the company had conducted its negotiations by only working to reduce the union's demands. Their theory seemed to be "give them anything except money." The union was directing work in the plants. This time, in preparing the company's agenda and counterproposal, I rewrote the labor union contract, voiding contradictions and updating out of date clauses. The union's reaction was that "The company never before asked for anything. This is an unfair practice on your part." My approach was important because changes had become necessary. In this case, negotiators on both sides took notice of the proposed changes and offered proposals and counterproposals that established trust and credibility. This new style for working together stood the test of time in subsequent negotiations.

The negotiations process is the leavening force of an ongoing relationship, rather than a one-time conflict between two parties who may never contend with each other again. Because of individual approaches and differences in negotiating, we should address this study of the process as an art rather than a science. We will be looking at broad and general ways to work toward solutions, always open to question and flexible adaptation. There will be road signs but no road maps. No two negotiating sessions are ever the same, no matter how often the parties have met across the table. Opponents change and adapt to the stances and values of those they represent.

We can perhaps best describe, or picture, the process as a sort of gradual spiral that moves forward—or in other directions, depending on the successive outcomes of negotiations—each time the parties reach a new agreement.

The process of negotiations can best be envisioned as a four-part activity: *preparation, drama, closing,* and *follow-up*. Of these, I believe that preparation is clearly the most important. A thorough preparation can become a major contributing factor to successful conclusion of negotiations: on a scale of 100 percent I would assign not less that 40 percent to preparation. Once prepared as well as the circumstances allow, the actual negotiation, or as I prefer to call this part, the drama, takes place. I have allotted this part no more than 20 percent. While this is the aspect of the process that gets most of the public attention, as well as the bulk of the written material that makes up the "how to's" on the market, the ability to be patient and persistent in working toward one's goals permeates the drama at the table. Closing, or wrapping up the agreements reached during the drama, and the follow-up to make the agreements work as they were intended to, each demand a 15 per cent value. Time and trust best describe this importance. While you may feel that your opponent means well, as you start to finalize the agreements that you believed were mutually agreed, you may find that the time you spent in preparation, negotiating, and bargaining have been wasted because of misunderstanding. This points to the need to obtain specific, explicit, written agreements as the bargaining process evolves. Write down what you both agree on and have that interim agreement initialed before you proceed so that when you have closed, you will be able to put together an agreement that can be written and signed that fulfills the mutual understandings. Once you have an agreed document, you must make sure that both parties live up to the signed agreement. Your opponent, and cosigner may well be a trustworthy person, but may not be the individual responsible for administering that agreement. Experience has demonstrated that what often takes place in contract administration replays the Bismarckian maxim that one should not

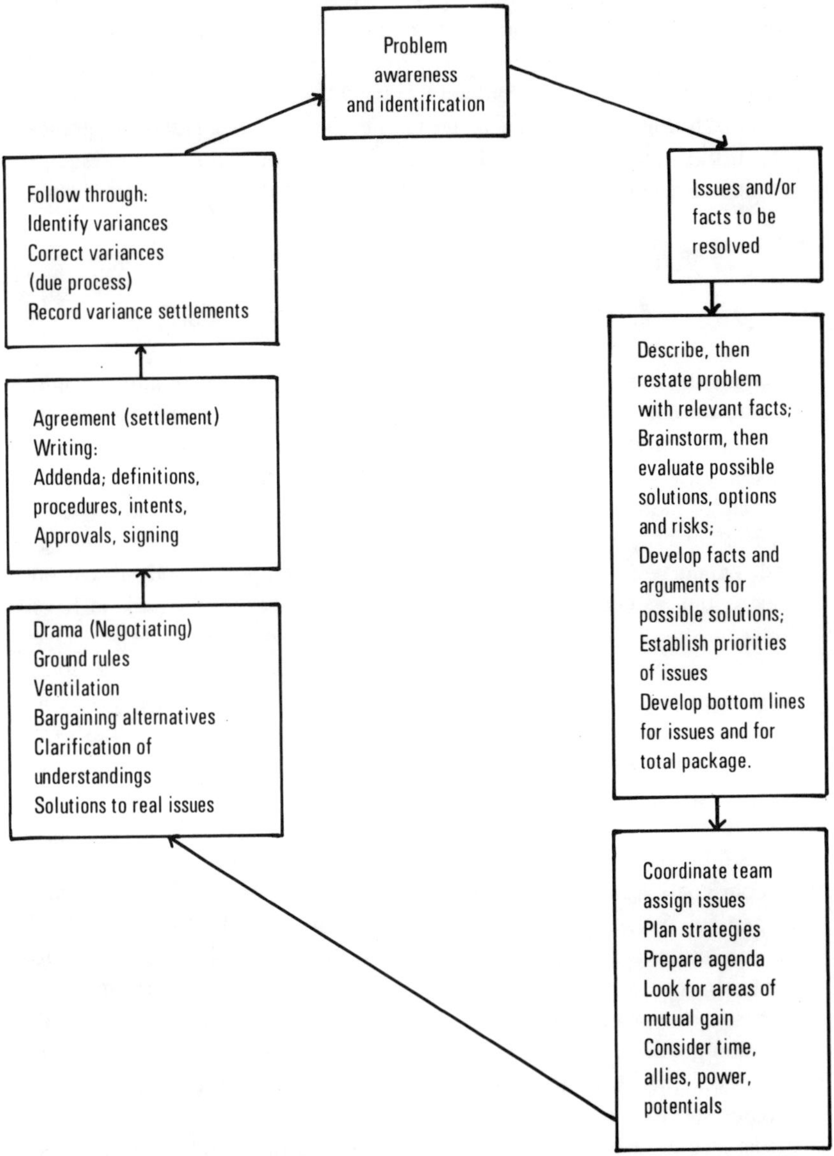
Problem awareness and identification
Issues and/or facts to be resolved
Describe, then restate problem with relevant facts; Brainstorm, then evaluate possible solutions, options and risks; Develop facts and arguments for possible solutions; Establish priorities of issues Develop bottom lines for issues and for total package.
Coordinate team assign issues Plan strategies Prepare agenda Look for areas of mutual gain Consider time, allies, power, potentials
Drama (Negotiating) Ground rules Ventilation Bargaining alternatives Clarification of understandings Solutions to real issues
Agreement (settlement) Writing: Addenda; definitions, procedures, intents, Approvals, signing
Follow through: Identify variances Correct variances (due process) Record variance settlements

expect a country (administrator, in our context) to honor agreements that are against its national interests. Administrators tend to see themselves as rulers and interpreters. They will, if unopposed, feel free to interpret sections of agreements in order to expand their personal bureaucracies. Without follow-up by either of the parties, misunderstandings are perpetrated, intentions are perverted, and goodwill goes down the drain. Again, all the time spent in preparation, negotiation and bargaining may have been wasted. Trust is fine, but constant vigilance is necessary to maintain it. The major steps in the negotiating process are illustrated above.

Problem Awareness and Identification

Goals and objectives must be determined long before negotiations begin. If you are not fully aware of what you *hope* to attain at the negotiation meetings you will not do well. When establishing your goals, it usually makes sense to set them at a level higher than you intend to settle. It is advisable, in nearly every negotiating situation to propose extra problems for settlement, proposals that have little or no chance of passing and ones with which you have little concern. The more proposals you present on your initial agenda—assuming that, on the surface, they appear to have some substance and can be made to sound reasonable—the more you have to "give" away. These extras give you maneuvering room at the table, make your opponent look good when you give them up, and may give you more of an opportunity to be persuasive later when you have to push for something you require.

Your Goals and Needs

Your goals are the product of your needs. Needs must be stated in terms of particulars such as services, contract terms and specifications, alternatives, costs, methods of payment and so forth. Should you be unable to establish your needs in precise terms, you will find that your ability to carry out the negotiations will be restricted. The lack of specificity in describing your needs will make it difficult to write a tightly-worded agreement, which ultimately will give rise to administrative difficulties. Having specific needs as the foundation for your goals will give you a better base to set your aspirations high and keep them high. Your success in negotiations will result from maintaining a high level of expectation, which can be kept that way with good preparation.

Setting goal objectives is the result of defining needs and creating high

The advantages to using a team include: the availability of supportive technical expertise; the possibility of developing more strategy options; the availability of more feedback from participants as well as pooling of information and impressions; and having worked within the group mandate, a broader base from which to sell negotiation results to the group (assuming that team unity has been effective). Team disadvantages include: the difficulty of preventing inadvertent leaks; the possibilities of individual disagreements over strategies, proposals and concessions (we are dealing with physicians, remember); the time necessary to prepare properly, to orient the team, and to sit at the negotiating table; and the Machiavellian propensity of an opponent to divide and conquer by encouraging team disagreements.

Implementation for Goal Preparedness - Research

Research probably will develop along several tracks. There will be the digging to make the case for getting the opponent to understand and negotiate for your goals. There will be the review of notes from previous negotiations, to learn the patterns and approaches used by both parties, *i.e.*, proposals made, pressures exerted, tactics used, credibility and authority to come to agreement, administration of past agreements, etc. There will have to be an assessment of the bargaining power of both parties—the weaknesses and strengths of each.

From the broad reach of suggested research, it should be obvious that being prepared for negotiations requires much more than understanding your own goals and expectations. By packaging your objectives into an agenda that tells your opponent what it is that you are seeking, you have taken a first step. But, in developing that agenda, you must also frame it with the understanding that it is not etched in stone—that concessions, alterations and withdrawals will have to be made while striving for agreement on as many of your goals as possible. With this work behind you, you will be prepared, during the negotiations, to act rather than to react, a position in which unprepared negotiators often find themselves.

Fact and data collection

Having established and clarified goals that are realistic and reasonably attainable, research should get underway immediately. State those objectives as questions—what, why or why not, when, how, etc. Then, because in many situations you will need time to dig for answers, look around for people to get the answers for you. This is not as difficult as it may first seem. Innumerable sources are available. But you have to find them. If statistical data is needed for backup, it can be found in libraries, government agencies, and various periodicals. Particularly, if negotiations will be with a government agency or with a government contractor, they can be used as a source to give their own data under freedom of information requests. Such requests should be as specific as possible, and should ask for as much of the backup material that went into the final data results.

A little-used source for data, close to your professional home, is the medical society, county, state and national, specialty and/or sub-specialty, as well as the various hospital associations. Quite often, depending upon the level that you first approach, and because they are seldom asked to assist in negotiations preparation, you are given a negative response. Ask them to ask the next higher organizational level for the answers to your questions. In situations requiring approach to the AMA, ask for their library information department. When given specific information requests, these people are among the most helpful people you can find.

What you do with the information that accumulates will be up to you, either as an individual negotiator or as a team specialist. You will find, quite often, that the answers you receive will raise many new questions. When this happens, you will have to go back to your sources or look for new ones.

Checking the history

Facts and data collection, as noted, are only part of your preparation. When researching the history of previous negotiations between the parties, start with the notes of those meetings. You will be looking for:

- Types and sources of factual information used by both parties, especially those sources used by the opponent;
- How the facts were presented by the parties and how credible they were at the time of presentation, as well as how they held up under discussion and questioning;
- Personality quirks of the negotiators, attitudes and apparent value systems of opponent negotiators especially if they will be across the table during this negotiations;
- Personal needs such as acceptance, a feeling of worth, and security, should be considered. Concessions to these intagibles will cost you nothing but can influence the outcome of a negotiation;

- Dependence of the parties upon written policies, regulations, rules, budgets, practices, etc., to reinforce stand-pat or seemingly less than rational positions (bureaucratic inertia);
- Use of time or other pressures;
- Flexibility in seeking rational and mutual solutions to the problems presented—or inflexibility, stubbornness, and unwillingness to take any position other than the ones brought to the table, to the point of impasse and the means required to resolve such impasses;
- Use of outside resources of influence to promote movement or acquiescence by either party; etc.

Having checked out how your opponents have operated in the past, you must do what you can to update that information about their representatives who will face you for the current negotiations. Knowing as much as you can about the person or people who will sit across from you will make it less difficult to devise strategies for your meetings. Their weaknesses, if you can determine them, will become a source of power for you. Based on their history (from past notes) and the current information you have collected, make a list of what you have learned:

- What are the weak spots? Will flattery work; will position or social relationships make him, or them, move carefully?
- Will the opponent be subject to public, political or private pressure? Who are the people who can be counted upon to assist you if things get tough?
- Does your opponent have a deadline or other pressure hanging over him that can be used to pressure him toward a decision?

Planning Strategies

Repetition in a variety of forms is inherent in negotiations. Foresight and flexibility are necessary to manipulate the emphasis that is placed on agenda items and to make reasonable concessions. Motives for negotiating must be carefully examined in order to formulate your minimum needs and your potential major concessions. Strategies should be planned, early in the negotiations, to develop a spirit of cooperative endeavor. Trust and credibility are cornerstones to mutually satisfactory settlements. Through the judicious use of questions that seek clarification of an opponent's real needs you demonstrate a sincere interest in his needs, and stroke his ego. However, while expressing your interest in your opponent's positions, care should be taken to establish bases for your own interests. This can be done by talking about the similarities and mutuality of both sets of goals as contrasted by their apparent differences. Opponents have a tendency to ignore arguments that appear to oppose their positions, mindsets, and instructions. To avoid hardening such attitudes, plan to understate the less desirable aspects of what you are proposing while at the same time stressing the similarities of both sides' goals. For physicians, no matter what the personal or group goals may be, financial aggrandizement will be the core issue but aspects of patient care will be and should be the leading argument. The problem faced by the physician negotiator will always be the framework within which to include this issue.

Use clear and concise language to emphasize the benefits your opponents will receive by accepting your demands. As the pros and cons of the potential solutions come alive for him, plan to finish the discussion with your most persuasive arguments. He'll remember these statements and they should be the ones that have the soundest basis for leading to a mutually satisfactory solution.

When planning strategies, remember that negotiations usually can be classified into two general situations. One category is where you or your services are needed. The other aspect is where you are in the position of promoting or selling yourself or your services in competition with others. These two sides of the coin, are not always mutually exclusive because, in today's health care market, competition for your needed services often exists.

Where your services are in demand, the better strategy may be to start with high demands. Experience seems to favor negotiators who begin by asking for more and apparently limiting what they are prepared to offer in return for the following reasons:

- By proposing what appear to be excessive subjects for discussion, the negotiator puts himself in the position of developing opportunities for clarifying his knowledge of the opponent's options and expectations;
- High expectations exhibit firm conviction on the part of the proposer;
- Initial high or excessive proposals have a tendency to put a dent in an opponent's expectations;

- By proposing a large number of not unreasonable issues, the negotiator lets the opponent know that he expects both fair treatment without exploitation; and
- With a large number of proposals for consideration, a negotiator gives himself the opportunity to make concessions that will gratify the opponent's desire for both accomplishment and control of his results.

However, be careful when planning and using such a grandiose "gimme" strategy. You can put your opponent in the position of becoming hard-nosed or uninterested if you fail to carefully communicate that you are not going into the negotiations with an unreasonable or rigid attitude. One idea that can, and usually does, tend to backfire is the characterization of proposals as "non-negotiable." Be prepared to let your opponent know that you may be willing to modify your expectations in order to come to a mutually satisfactory solution.

When the situation changes and you have to convince your opponent to sit down and talk with you about services that you are selling, you need a different approach. You have to capture your opponent's interest. Your best approach may be to stress the benefits that will accrue to him and to the patients from the utilization of your special talents. Once you have his attention and interest you are ready to discuss terms and conditions. Threats should not be a part of your strategy to get an opponent to the negotiating table unless you are prepared to carry them out. Threats will create hostility and color future relationships. Promises that will be kept, as well as offers to discuss the use of your services, have a tendency to create a more favorable feeling on the part of the person that you are trying to impress.

Establishing the mood

Each negotiation develops its own tone and direction. The purpose of developing a strategy each time you prepare to sit with an opponent is to set up a basis for influencing that tone and/or direction. Whether you come to the table with a friendly, antagonistic, or nonchalant attitude—your tone—or whether you act pressured or relaxed—and your direction—will set the stage for the way your opponent will react to your proposals. Through the planned use of alternative proposals, in effect, unforeseen and imaginative approaches to what appear to be mundane solutions, you may put your opponent off balance and be better able to press for your goals.

Plan your strategies so that they will not become a straitjacket. Take a hard look at both sides of the issue; at the issues that will work for or against you, and think through to the possible effects that your proposals may have upon both your opponent and any third parties (public, insurors, etc.) to create resistance. You will have to reduce or remove that resistance by working on your opponent's needs. Develop a strategy that will make his needs work for your own goals rather than against you. How you implement your basic strategy will be covered in later chapters.

As a negotiator you should have a range of strategies as well as personality strengths from which to draw. Today's successful strategy may prove quite innappropriate tomorrow. The negotiator who learns to adapt to changing or unexpected situations and flexes his approaches will usually come closest to achieving his goals. The more resourceful you are, the better you will be able to deal with the wide range of unpredictable situations you will meet.

Risk

Making assumptions is an easily overlooked but major risk taken by many negotiators. The risk lies in not checking out ideas or presumptions that, for a variety of reasons, are taken for granted. The variables that result from a negotiator's subjective evaluations of either his preliminary views resulting from his preparation, or his estimates of situations as the negotiations proceed, should be questioned and requestioned in order to be properly assessed. A negotiator must avoid, at all costs, taking a static—or self-satisfied—view of what is always an extremely dynamic process. Questioning one's subjective responses to an opponent's negotiating style can build the bridges that one needs to get from assumed perceptions to the more real world of negotiations.

Regulations

When considering potential risk, penalties that may be assessed should be checked out. Penalties may be associated with laws or regulations that limit what may be attempted. Often laws and regulations contradict each other. These visible differences can sometimes be used to open different corridors to problem-solving. However, you must appreciate that each bureaucracy follows its interpretation of a law and ignores anyone else's. This is where the evaluation of risk comes in—is the fight worth the cost, in both time and money? One thought to keep in mind about regulations—they are too often interpreted in ways that change the regulation as it was originally written. Interpretive memoranda, special letters within the agency, and, most misleading of all, the verbal interpretations that exponentially confuse issues as they are passed from one officeholder to the next with each new interpreter taking what is told as gospel so the real regulations don't have to be learned and read. The risk, particularly in preparation, lies in accepting someone's sayso rather than going to the written source. Written and published regulations may enable you to redirect misinterpretations. You will at least have a base from which to negotiate, because unless an interpretation has been publically announced, it should be contested as someone's private view and not that applicable to the public it is supposed to serve.

Hospital bylaws

Written hospital bylaws are often overlooked, perhaps because of their proximity in both inter- and intra-organization negotiation. Too often, those who should know the rules under which all physicians accredited to a hospital-medical staff have bound themselves in order to have privileges on that staff, do not. Then, should disciplinary action or fulfillment of certain committee or other responsibility be required, people react cavalierly. Most of the time such reaction is without any base. The bylaws often have not been thoroughly reviewed by the majority of the staff. The risk here is that it is too easy to put one's foot in one's mouth by taking a position that would not have been taken if the speaker had reread the bylaws. As noted earlier, rules, regulations, and any written material for handling relationships with people should be given more than a glance—read them closely to discover the areas that are not being adhered to, are being abused, or, at the very least, areas in which you may find a handle to redirect the negotiations more to your favor.

The time crunch

Misuse of time is another risk that is often overlooked until it is too late. Physicians and administrator are busy people. But some professionals merely project the image of being busy to use time as a weapon. Time is usually negotiable. Opponents may try to impose deadlines. You may want to have a deadline. But time is not always as firmly fixed as opponents may try to make you believe. Be aware of how time allotted to the negotiation process is being used—often against your better interests. It can put you under pressure to make quick decisions that you regret later. If, through delaying tactics such as procrastination in producing substantial answers to questions, your opponent appears to be avoiding decision-making, don't show that you are upset. If he is trying to squeeze you into the time corner to make a decision in his favor., suggest that "because we seem to be getting on so well and so close to agreement, let's meet again tomorrow and iron out the little differences." If, however, you want an agreement, you have to be willing to insist on decisions by a certain time. At the beginning of a negotiation deadlines appear to be reachable. But as talking goes on and becomes repetitious, time passes and the negotiations become mired and lose momentum. Deadlines can be imposed or insisted upon to get things moving, but make sure you gauge their results.

If you are negotiating with nine-to-five opponents, they will want to have the meetings during working hours. Administrators may not like to meet too often outside those hours. But, as physicians who are used to working at least half-again as much as the nine-to-fivers, you are busiest during those same hours with patient care—office hours, or meeting other patient needs. You might suggest meeting after six o'clock or on weekends. This will not always work to your complete advantage—because of time pressures on the other side—but you may be able to balance the meeting times to get more time for patient care.

Bluffs and threats

Negotiators who want to throw their weight around, either for their own ego-enhancement or as part of a strategy planned to buttress a weak bargaining position, may bluff or threaten. Bluffs are positions that usually are not backed by facts or logic, but that may lead one's opponent to assume that the backup is available. A bluff that leads to an unprovable assumption may be a feint, an outright lie, or an intended misrepresentation of fact. Anytime you believe you are being bluffed, question your assumptions and your opponent—get to the truth of the issue. Lost bluffs negate the user's credibility and make opponents leary of later legitimate negotiating tactics. And credibility, once lost or damaged in the other side's opinion, is difficult to regain. Bluffs and threats should be used very, very carefully, if at all, and, if you do, be sure you are capable of carrying them out. The risk of being caught in a bluff, a non-performable threat, an outright lie, or some form of misrepresentation, and the negative effect that such deceit can have on one's ability to successfully negotiate is serious. Keep such usage out of your negotiating body of guidelines.

Bargaining in good faith

One of the cornerstones of negotiating behavior is the expectation of reciprocal good faith. This can be an insidious risk. If you are negotiating honestly and openly, and your opponent is responding in a similar manner, negotiations through concessions and mutual understandings should progress satisfactorily. Verbal agreements are made. Then the opponent or his attorney offer to put the agreements in writing for signature. When you get the final document, it clashes with your recollection of what you had agreed to. What has occurred is not necessarily a reversal of good faith or intent. Rather it emphatically proves that the semantics of agreement require something more permanent than verbalization without clarification. The best way to promote understanding and clarity for mutual nongrievous administration of an agreement is to make written agreements as the negotiations proceed. Such notes need not be in the final language, but should be in such form that both parties understand the agreement, making last minute revisions unnecessary. These gradual consolidations of understandings become risk-reducers and, in a way, insurors of more than superficial good faith from those who come into a negotiations with less than sincere intentions.

No one's infallible

Finally, a reminder that one of the biggest and easiest risks that a physician too often takes is assuming that he knows or understands what is being discussed or proposed. All assumptions should be checked out. Question for clarification; restate for verification; ask for proof even if doubt is minimal. Don't assume, please.

Power

"Power" is one of those words that the expositors of the negotiating process like to use in their discussions. What they are presenting is a negotiator's ability, by whatever means, to achieve objectives by influencing opponents, or motivating those opponents to be reasonably agreeable to the negotiator's objectives. Power in negotiations is a form of pressure that is more often perceived than actualized. It is important to appreciate that, regardless of how powerful one negotiator perceives an opponent to be, such negotiating power is not all-encompassing. Absolute power seldom is available to one side because its possession and use are often formless and flexible.

Power in negotiating comes in a variety of effects. Physicians come to the table powered by reputation, training, and the ability to alleviate or cure most medical malfunctions. Hospital administrators and boards of directors exercise power by using laws and fiscal responsibilities as their levers with entrepeneurial associates, as well as a framework within which to provide patient care. They also invoke the *respondeat superior* doctrine in their employer-employee relationships. Insurors, both governmental and private, blatantly use the power of money, either to be paid or withheld from payment, to enforce their positions. Potential competitors, as peers or in some less-than-peer relationship, may try to effect change or compliance through use of the law, nitpicking through some sort of grievance process, and/or pressure alliances.

Everyone who is party to a negotiation has some power to bring to the negotiating table. How that power is perceived by an opponent, as well as how a negotiator uses the power available to him, will help determine how well either party achieves its goals for a negotiation. Neither party would be at a negotiating table if each did not have or need something that the other party needed or wanted. How well those needs and wants are satisfied can be enhanced by:

- Reward and/or punishment—depends on how well one reads an opponent during negotiation and what is most likely to influence the opponent as an individual and as a negotiating representative.
- Knowledge—depends on how well one can control the flow of information at the table and how credible it is (we're back to preparation, research, and objectives development). Expertise and experience gain respect, another form of power.
- Time, effort, and commitment—patience can work for you. Willingness to work toward reasonable goals, flexibly, without being taken advantage of, can influence an opponent.
- Competition/uncertainty—includes willingness to introduce and/or accept risk; taking a positive stand on principle, knowing that you may deadlock if your opponent does not agree to some variant of that principle. An insoluble deadlock can bring a negotiation to the point where raw power is brought into play.
- Research/preparation/skill—base and backup for knowledge. The more effort that is expended to substantiate your premises and objectives, to anticipate your opponent's posits and reactions, and to gather supportable quantitative analyses and facts, the greater your bargaining power.

- Bureaucracies—they can be used to support a position, argue that laws, rules, regulations, policies, budgets, and precedents do (or do not, depending upon a particular situation) reinforce your negotiating stance. If your research develops supportable and confusing practices or interpretations, lock on to the one that is most favorable to your position and that may call for higher-up intercession.
- Relations with an opponent—friendly relations can ease tenseness during tough negotiating sessions. Friendship should not be used to demand an advantage from an opponent—someday that favor will have to be returned, with interest.
- Supports and endorsements—your position may be given greater legitimacy if it is supported by people that your opponent perceives as having bargaining power or influence. Having the stated approval of one's medical staff peers can influence an aggressive administrator. Political support can be of help in dealing with bureaucrats. However, such support should be used infrequently and with care. The negotiator who depends upon name-dropping alone—without the full support of proper preparation, skill, and timing—will be less successful in achieving goals.
- Reputation—last, but certainly not least, your own standing—in the community, within the profession—as an expert, as a professional, as a person concerned with the patient's well-being (and with their potential vocal support), if perceived or recognized by your opponent, will enhance your negotiating status and power.

Recognize power for what it may be, and use it carefully. Don't assume that your opponent is holding all the cards. Curiosity, innovative thinking, and patience, should be relied upon to go beyond the perception of an opponent's apparent power. Probe, evaluate the potential risks, discover where the power that you believe is there comes from and how it may be used against you, and work out, if possible, a counter. Remember that in all your preparation, you are working toward a positive result—the goals and objectives that you have set for this negotiation. Remember, too, that the strategies and tactics, the perceptions and evaluations that you have made about your opponent, perhaps even your goals and objectives, are not fixed in concrete—that flexibility (within reason) and patience are the name of the game. As you both develop your positions, progress will come from the reactions of both parties, and the way those reactions are interpreted and met. Relate to what is going on across the table, and, somehow (I know that this is easier to say to you than it may be for you to practice) *be comfortable* with whatever it is that you are doing at that negotiation.

Preparing the Agenda

After establishing your goals and objectives, collecting information to verify your positions and those of your opponent, and planning your basic strategies, you are ready to prepare an agenda. Too often, opponents assume that, because they both know, in general terms, what the negotiations will be about, that all they have to do is sit down and get to work. If they have been in close contact for some time, that may well be the case. However, even if you and your opponent are good friends and believe that the negotiations will be a friendly discussion with the results fairly well predetermined, you are advised to prepare a written agenda.

An agenda need not be an elaborate statement of goals and their reasons. Your agenda should be a list of the topics and mutual problems that you want to discuss and for which you seek satisfactory solutions. The items on an agenda, stated in very general terminology, should not necessarily be in either ascending or descending order of importance—it is better to mix them up. In any case as you get started the order in which the problems are taken up will be a matter of mutual consent. Your opponent may look upon a prepared agenda as a means of attacking your premises if he is of a mind to obstruct the course of the negotiations. He may try to insist on following only his agenda, completing and agreeing on each item before going on to the next. This must be avoided. If you can't reach an agreement on the agenda, suggest third party assistance.

Your agenda is a part of your overall strategy. With it, you are giving your opponent his first real idea of your goals for this negotiation. Every agenda should contain a "saver" note: that you reserve the right to add other subjects that may result from what the negotiations bring out. While you are offering your opponent an opportunity to clarify his pre-negotiation judgments about your goals, his agenda offers you the same opportunity. Together, the two agendas can be discussed and combined to make a single, general outline for the negotiations. Areas of mutual concern will quickly become evident. These can be the objects of immediate discussion, leaving those items that are not common to either agenda to be taken up later. Unless the mutual subjects are based upon emotionally subjective positions, negotiations should be able to get off to a good start, developing a momentum for mutual gain and trust for the more difficult items that are important to each side.

Problem definition

The agenda rationalizes problem definition and explication, and the negotiations take off from that point. The common agenda or your written agenda bring the discussions back on track when they are wandering, appear to be bypassing some of your more important items, or are moving into an impasse situation . . . " That's an interesting suggestion and it deserves more discussion, but let's take another look at our proposal eight. . ."

An agenda may have some "red herrings"—apparently irrelevant issues put on the negotiating table either as tools to divert your attention from the real issues (these are uncovered either by questioning their usefulness to the opponent, or by ignoring them and moving on to something more productive to the real issues). Red herrings are important because they can give a negotiator maneuvering room if properly used. They become give-aways that cost you nothing because they are not important to your final needs. They make the opponent feel good in getting you to back off something he sees as a threat to a satisfactory conclusion to the negotiations, or they confuse the real issues and serve to overextend the time set aside for negotiating. "Patient care," that buzz-word that says so much and yet so little, can be a *raison d'etre* for both sides to lean on. If effectively presented in either a subjective (medically indicated by training and practice) or objective (cost-effective yet good for the patient) presentation, patient care can be a red herring.

An agenda tells an opponent why one is at the table. It is an indicator of motivations for the individuals who are negotiating—for themselves or for the parties that they represent. These factors include money (number one in most negotiations, regardless of the layers of moral or other justifications with which the agenda items are clothed), service, security (which can be either individual or collective), and self-importance. Discovering those motivations behind the formal agenda and playing to them or through them will help make you a better and more successful negotiator.

After the preparation, the next step is the drama. A poor performance at this stage can affect the outcome of the negotiations.

To help you feel comfortable with the recommendations in this book, we will use case study frameworks. The format will present background information from which you should determine how you would proceed if you were in that situation. Questions that you might be asking yourself appear in Appendix B. (Remember, there is no *one* way to handle negotiating situations. How you proceed is up to you. Your path through these cases is up to you—as long as you are *comfortable* with it.) It is strongly recommended that you not go to the back of the book until you have thought through and written out your plans or actions.

**** **** ****

Scenario I

Negotiating from a percentage contract to one more favorable

South Fork Medical Center is a 510 bed community hospital in a midwest metropolitan area. A previously successful and well-qualified administrator recently has been hired by the board of directors. He accepted the position and was designated the Executive Vice-president (EVP) of the hospital corporation. For the past three years the hospital has been approaching financial instability. The new EVP was hired, in part, because in his last position he successfully assisted in reversing the financial trouble of a similar medical institution.

In the course of becoming acquainted with his financial situation and problems, the EVP determined that the gross earnings of the hospital-based professionals, all of whom were in the hospital on gross revenue percentage agreements, averaged in excess of $136,000. When the EVP attempted to conduct a confidential survey of hospital-based physician earnings and other conditions of hospital service and remuneration current throughout the metropolitan area, he ran into resistance from his fellow administrators. They were either hesitant about admitting that they were not in complete control of their contractual arrangements or they were fearful that the eventual publication of the findings would put them into less attractive situations *vis-a-vis* their own hospital-based specialists. Following face-to-face visits with his fellow administrators and his promise to limit both the accumulation of data and the exchange of collected information to the chief executive officers (CEOs) with whom he met, everyone was assured of institutional anonymity and the survey was completed.

Survey results revealed that most hospital-based physician's earnings (gross) that were based upon percentages of departmental billings were, as expected, relatively and uniformly above published national averages for those specialties. Earnings appeared to be related in parallel to the size and gross operating receipts of the area hospitals. South Fork, as the third largest of the area hospitals, determined that its anesthesiologists were among the top earners in their specialty, radiologists second highest, and pathologists fourth among their peers. The EVP's study of the South Fork data disclosed diminishing profits from these three specialty areas, apparently from what he perceived to be the results of increases in operating costs—actually, in large part the result of union organizing and contracts of technicians and other hospital personnel, and the inflated costs of supplies and equipment modernization. His internal study also disclosed that because of these increased operating costs the professional's income had increased. The growing use of the specialty services was also noticed but not remarked upon by the EVP. Since an increasing percentage of the hospital census was coming from Medicare and Medicaid patients, the hospital was experiencing less than complete payments in relation to its billings from the Medicare carrier and the state welfare department.

The EVP, with the board's executive committee, after reviewing and discussing the survey results, decided that all professional percentage contracts with the hospital should be terminated and new agreements be negotiated, or imposed, as soon as possible. With full board approval, letters were sent to all hospital-based physicians giving notice of termination as required by the current contracts, and requesting negotiations to be conducted and completed during the notice period, to be held with the hospital's financial vice-president.

You are the president of the professional corporation that has had exclusive privileges for your specialties in South Fork Medical Center for the past ten years. All previous negotiations have been with the hospital administrator, and all have been settled with a handshake and covered by a short letter of understanding. You and your associates, as well as the other hospital-based specialists, have been surprised by the action taken by the hospital, particularly since no early warning was noticed. Your corporate attorney has never negotiated a hospital or any other personal service type contract and does not seem eager to begin with your situation.

What Are You Going To Do?

Using what you have been studying thus far, prepare for negotiations. Turn to Appendix B for a suggested course of action.

**** **** ****

Scenario II

Tweedeldum Hospital is a 196-bed hospital in a county seat in the center of a prosperous farming community. A number of small industries, several of which are units of larger corporations based elsewhere, furnish employment for members of the community. The board of directors (12) is headed by the president of the largest local bank, and includes the current chief of the medical staff. Members of the board have received copies of the report of the Joint Committee on Accreditation of Hospitals (JCAH) downgrading the hospital's accreditation to temporary, giving them 180 days to make major improvements. The JCAH inspection visit made it very clear that the hospital had to make many corrections to continue its accreditation. The inspectors told everyone what was required to meet the stricter expectations of JCAH. Neither the administrator nor the medical staff leadership has given the survey team much thought, since no warnings have ever been issued before.

Included among the shortcomings in hospital administration and quality control noted by the JCAH inspection team ascribed to the areas supervised by the hospital-based specialties were:

- A lack of medical quality control on any kind of a regular random-type review;
- No formal audits or overview of hospital-based specialty performance by bylaw-authorized committeess as set forth in the medical staff bylaws;
- An apparent lack of communication between the hospital-based specialites and the staff physicians, both through written and verbal means, pertaining to recommendations of pre- and post-operative situations and non-operative patients;
- Medical staff bylaws that were out-of-date, having never been updated to reflect current staff practices, authorities or responsibilities; and,
- An apparent hoarding of pertinent information concerning patient care that required attending physicians to request data needed for continued patient care.

Faced with this deadline to make corrections or lose accreditation, the board, under the firm direction of the chairman, has directed the administrator to rewrite the bylaws of both the board and the medical staff and to have the first drafts before the board at their next meeting—in 60 days. Included in those instructions was a recommendation to establish a full-time medical director who would be the permanent senior officer of the medical staff reporting to the administrator and also would be a member of the board of directors. In line with the developing law allocating the basic responsibility for hospital quality to boards of directors, the administrator was instructed to include means for the board to establish controls for setting, monitoring, and enforcing compliance with professional standards of quality care and patient safety.

The administrator quickly put together revised sets of bylaws with the help of the hospital attorney, an individual experienced in this field. Copies of both sets of bylaws were given to the board members for study, and to the executive committee of the medical staff. Both sets of bylaws clarified the authority and accountability of the hospital board of directors and established objectives for the functional divisions of the hospital. The proposed bylaws effectively subordinated the former independent and vaguely accountable medical staff to the managerial supervision of the board and its designated representative—the administrator. The medical staff bylaws specifically defined the expected purposes and responsibilities of committees for quality patient care. Included in the functional responsibilities for the medical staff organization were:

- Responsibilities for making recommendations to the board, through the administrator, for the establishment, maintenance and continuous improvement of medical professionalism;
- regular and consistent review, analysis and evaluation of the hospital and professional practices of medical staff members' quality of patient care;
- Regular periodic reports through the administrative channels to the board of attending physician's clinical performance relative to professional standards, with recommendations for implementation and enforcement of those standards as well as corrective action where required;
- Recommendations for appointments, including verification procedures, and reappointments to the medical staff with procedures for assuring and monitoring privileges;
- Exercising, through surveillance audits, discipline as required by the limited uthority delegated by the board while offering and observing objective due process;
- Working with the hospital administration and the board to plan and effectuate hospital aims to meet needs of the community;

- Supervising and maintaining ongoing continuing educational programs for practicing physicians and other hospital personnel to assure quality patient care;
- Assuring compliance of the medical staff with the bylaws rules, regulations and policies as published, as well as observing and commenting on compliance by all other areas of the hospital staff.

You are the Chief of Staff of the hospital medical staff, and your term runs out in two months. Rumors of the JCAH recommendations and intentions have been lowering physician morale while accentuating self-righteous indignation. Communication with the administrator has been friendly but very formal. Copies of the revised recommended bylaws have been delivered to you through the house mail with a note that approval by the medical staff is expected within three weeks.

What Are You Going To Do?

Using what you have been studying so far, what are your options? Will you negotiate? If yes, how will you prepare? Turn to Appendix B for a suggested course of action.

**** **** ****

Practice Negotiation Self-Critique

Check your preparation plans against the following factors:

1. Adequacy of preparation—analysis of hospital positions and bargaining power, expectation levels of both sides, analysis of potential settlement ranges, facts required for positions to be taken, counter arguments for expected hospital positions, and potential allies and enemies.
2. Underlying problems for hospital positions, your positions? Are these down on paper? Remember, you are looking for causes, basic problems, not symptoms.
3. Completeness of facts and information to assist you in reaching a mutually satisfactory solution.
4. Possible alternatives if you are unable to realize your stated goals. Or, are you trying to maintain something close to the *status quo?*

5. Preparation of a written agenda. Have you committed your priorities and bottom lines to another sheet of paper?

Having given yourself satisfactory answers to all the above, ARE YOU *COMFORTABLE* WITH YOUR PLANS?

5
NEGOTIATIONS DRAMA—ALL THE ACTS

It takes two to make a bargain.
It's a bad bargain where nobody gains.

English Proverb

The drama of the negotiation process—that's where interaction takes place. As with any drama, this stage of the process can be divided into a number of acts and scenes. In the beginning stages, the parties must arrive at agreements on such basic details as: agenda; locations, times and length of meetings; use of resource persons and/or size of negotiating teams; actual or potential deadlines; and, most important, each opponent's authority to negotiate and commit the institution or party that he represents. Act II, following the preliminaries, will advance the presentation of each party's problems and concerns, with the negotiators putting their justifications and potential solutions on the table, searching for hidden agenda and interests, and establishing the bases for solutions that will lead to mutual gain. Finally, in Act III will come negotiation and bargaining for mutually satisfactory solutions and agreement.

Unlike conventional drama, the scenes and acts will probably not be orderly and sequential. Disagreements and/or questions over agenda items can, and usually do, intervene in the conversations to precipitate temporary stalemates, which may require moving to another subject. This can maintain the rhythm and forward motion of the negotiations, giving the parties time either to restudy their information and their opponent's for that subject, finding possible avenues for agreement. Sometimes, in the course of working on an agenda item, one of the parties can inadvertantly make a remark that offers a quick and reasonable solution to another item of equal concern. With that, the current conversation is postponed and the new issue is discussed and probably settled at some future negotiation.

As the drama proceeds, agreements are made. No one of these agreements is final or binding upon the parties until both agree that they have covered everything they came to the negotiations for, and all the interim agreements are brought together into a single document. But, the possibility always exists that agreement on all agenda items may not be accomplished in a negotiation, yet interim agreements are useful to both parties. In such cases the opponents can decide to execute only those points they have resolved while admitting that major issues remain to be settled.

Interim agreements are the backbone of effective negotiations. However, too often such agreements are not completely understood, or the mental pictures of semantic presentations have different meanings to opposing parties than were intended by either. "So, we agree," "Can we consider that out of the way?" and similar quotes will abound between the first and last meetings. But what do the opposite parties really understand? Don't depend upon what you think you heard! Put it into a memo! The limited time that it will take you to write out your understanding of what you have just agreed to will be well spent. Any difference of opinion as to specifics of the latest item to be put aside as settled should be cleared up immediately. If you—or your opponent—take a number of understandings for granted, when you come to the final agreement and enumerate all the "good things" that both feel make for a win/win result, you will discover that neither of you agreed to what the other thought he had. Then negotiations have to resume, with tempers and questions of good faith and credibility interfering and possibly affecting the final result. Commitments should be made in writing. Each initialed piece of paper becomes part of a personal involvement in the outcome of the negotiations. Make the movement to final settlement flow smoothly. You will be glad that you did.

Steps to Agreement

Let's picture the stages that can occur for a single issue. As noted earlier, these phases may not take place uninterruptedly. Other issues or temporary stalemates may interrupt the flow. However, the pattern is eventually restarted and continued.

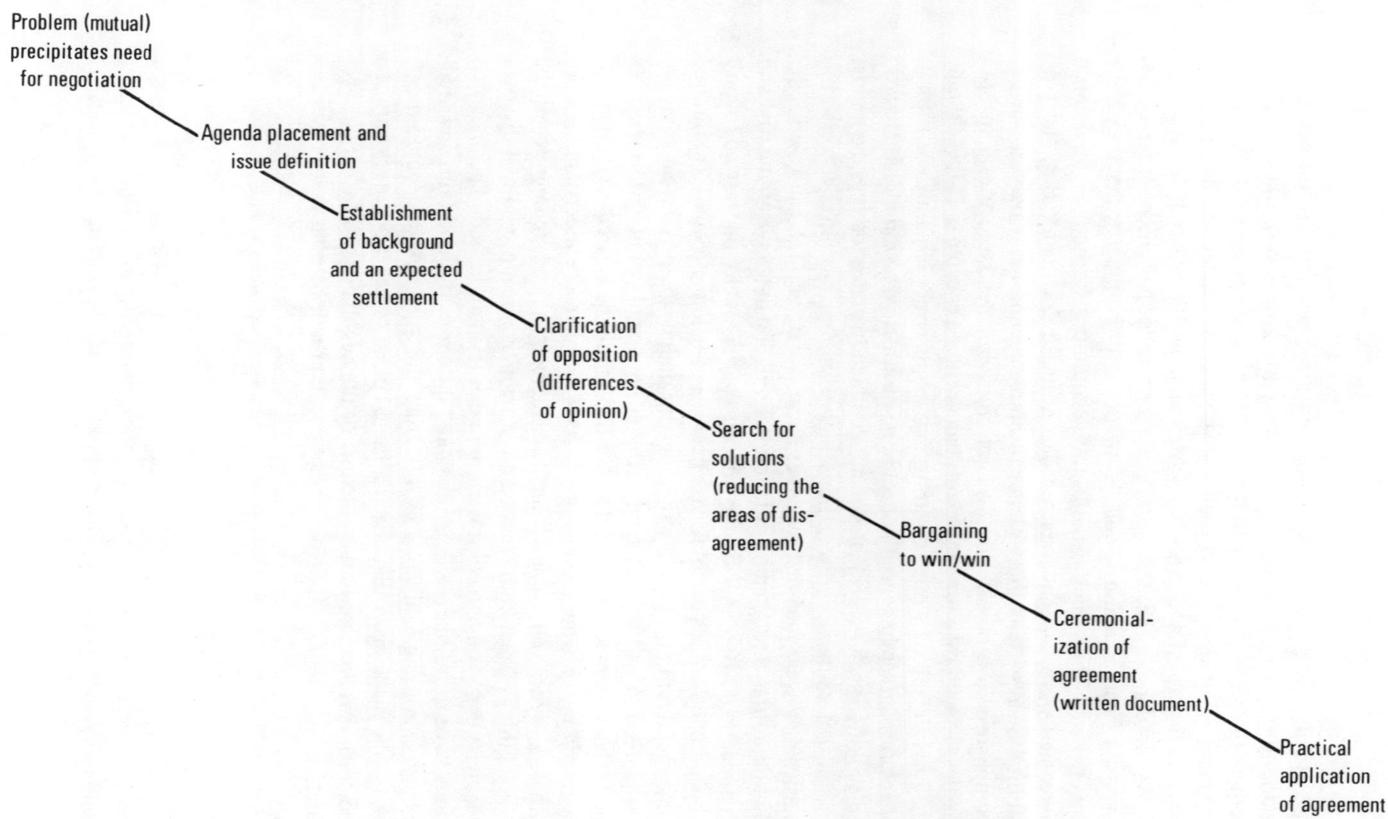

Problem (mutual) precipitates need for negotiation
Agenda placement and issue definition
Establishment of background and an expected settlement
Clarification of opposition (differences of opinion)
Search for solutions (reducing the areas of disagreement)
Bargaining to win/win
Ceremonialization of agreement (written document)
Practical application of agreement

We usually negotiate in order to effect or oppose change. Change, unfortunately, tends to upset opponents. It disrupts the complacency of routine and habit patterns, and it demands that one adapt to unexpected demands on the normal, or what has become accepted, practice. But change is inevitable and essential to improving and development. *Flexibility*—the ability to adapt to changing situations—is most necessary for the survival of your practice. For example, the imposition of DRGs will change your practice in terms of patients, hospitals, utilization reviews, and potential malpractice allegations. By looking to the future and the options that may be available with clear thinking, you will be able to mesh with that future. If you can roll with the changes in attitudes that the times and competition are forcing, you will stay ahead. Emotions have no part—or should have no part—in evaluating and choosing those options. How you negotiate for your best interests is up to you. Few will do it for you to your best advantage.

The tone of a negotiations often will become evident during the first meeting. An earlier attitude of friendliness and cordiality may be dissipated by the manner in which the demand for negotiation was proposed. If that happens, put aside those negative feelings. Most opponents appreciate a cooperative approach—and your friendly attitude may help them into a similar stance. This does *not* mean that you are obligating yourself to offer or make immediate concessions in order to justify your deportment. But exercising your self control, having a friendly approach to the meetings, and engaging in small talk may help both parties keep the flow of communications open and eventually assist in developing understandings as you go along. Be friendly and cooperative, but also be firm. You'll find that these traits give you an air of calm strength that will enhance your bargaining position.

Structure your handling of the discussions, proposals and counterproposals in direct and definite terms. For instance, instead of immediately going into long explanations of the ways in which your position differs from your opponent's, first suggest the ways in which the two positions may be similar. By emphasizing similarities instead of differences, you make the two positions appear closer than they may really be. The importance of timing this method of putting counterproposals or restating an opponent's statements cannot be overemphasized. For one thing, the positive approach will not lead your opponent into thinking that he could have squeezed you a little more if he had negotiated somewhat harder.

Why Negotiate?

Hospital administrators under cost pressures—and which one isn't—may try to be casual in their lead-in to the reasons for negotiating. Renegotiation of an expired agreement is reasonable. In rewriting a current contract, however, the administrator will probably try to include more restrictive clauses on the theory that proliferating medical subspecialization and expensive technological change and increasing income-source regulation are putting the hospital in a variety of squeezes. Be wary of proposed new language that you haven't had an opportunity to review carefully. Don't comment, either positively or negatively, when it is put on the table. Ask for a detailed explanation, the reasons for putting this language on the table, what it is supposed to accomplish, and how it will affect you, your work in the hospital, and your relationships with your peers and other hospital personnel. Then recess the meeting, take it home with you, and think about what you've been told. Too often developing a new solution to what someone visualizes as a real or imagined problem creates new problems, usually to your detriment.

With about half of the hospital-based physicians working without formal contracts or with only handshakes sealing their hospital arrangements, administrators are trying to tie hospital-based doctors to contracts. Without one, they think they have no control of what goes on in their institution. Several approaches may be used. The administrator may verbalize the hospital's need for a formal document in order to better define relationships within the hospital, either because of the tendency for patients' litigiousness—sliding the primary blame toward you—or because of the increasing tightfistedness of third-party reimbursers. They may quote apparent inconsistencies that have come to light because of changes in corporate bylaws, medical staff bylaws, rules, regulations or procedures; or new policies that may be required because of various mandatory, concurrent or retrospective audits. New JCAH recommendations—how do these coordinate or conflict with recommendations of your specialty society, if at all?; changes in state, OSHA, other licensing or regulatory agency laws or rules, such as hospital reclassification may also be presented as reasons for putting you under contract or changing existing contract clauses. Again, ask for a detailed explanation of why these proposed changes are on the table, what they are supposed to accomplish, how they will affect you with your work in the hospital, your peers, and other hospital personnel. Then, recess the meeting, take the proposal home with you, and think about what you have been told.

Finally, you may be told that departmental administrative problems show a need for formal contracts. Your lack of administrative efficiency may be cited. You might be accused of treating hospital personnel under your supervision differently than hospital policy allows, or of being too lenient with time off, or of arranging pay scales and personal bonuses that aren't in keeping with other departments, or of not following hospital purchasing procedures.

If you do not now have a contract, and the administrator is trying to tie you to one, discuss at length how these proposals may affect your relationship with the hospital, what aspects of your service within the hospital need alteration, and why these changes can't be handled the same way as previous rule or policy changes. Ask the administrator who harps on the necessity of a formal, legal document why none of the other members of the medical staff require contracts in order to bring their patients into the hospital for treatment. Insist upon a complete enumeration of duties and responsibilities. Some administrators tend to ease contractors and employees into additional duties and responsibilities step by step without offering payment or appreciation in return. (If you are going through contract *re*negotiation, follow the earlier suggestions—question, listen, requestion, recess, and consider.)

Planning Your Negotiating Sessions

While no two negotiations will be exactly the same—negotiators, problems, conditions and situations surrounding the problems discussed always being subject to change—they will generally conform to a pattern. That pattern will look something like the following:

- First session will:
  - Establish the negotiating climate
  - Establish a foundation of principles
  - Establish negotiating schedules
  - Establish negotiating routines
  - Exchange and explain proposals
- Second session will:
  - Clarify the purpose of specific proposals
  - Establish the basic principles of each proposal

- -- Explain, in detail, arguments for each proposal
- -- Avoid, if possible, disclosure of positions on own proposals
- Third session will:
  - -- Prepare groundwork for own counterproposals
  - -- Work opponent discussion of his proposals around to own counterproposals
- Succeeding sessions will:
  - -- Prepare groundwork for own proposals
  - -- Search for areas of agreement in principle
  - -- Work to positive understandings of areas of agreement or disagreement of proposals
  - -- Offer counterproposals where there are disagreements, discuss to agreement or impasse
  - -- Work out impasses
  - -- Make written record of agreements in principle
  - -- Put all agreements in writing for final agreement
  - -- Sell, and get concurrence on agreement from principals

With the pattern of the negotiating drama in mind, you will need to prepare in advance for each negotiating session to be sure all items that you want to discuss are, in fact, put on the table.

Negotiations can take place in an atmosphere where one or both sides in effect come out swinging for a fight to the finish, but this approach is not recommended or necessary. The parties can subdue animosity and negotiate to conclude mutually satisfactory solutions.

To insure a civil atmosphere some details should be clarified at the *first meeting*. That is the time to establish ground rules for:

- Avoiding discussions that do not lead to mutually satisfactory agreements;
- Using language that both sides understand for the purpose, effect and background of proposals. This includes the mechanics proposed to effectuate the proposals, to be sure that the proposal is workable and fair to both sides;
- Setting up times and locations of meetings. Because, as a practicing physician, you serve patients in the hospital or office, time for nego-

tiations may have to be found apart from the busier periods in the work day. Also, while each side has other duties to perform, and is interested in concluding the negotiations as quickly as possible, time must be made available to study proposals and counteroffers;

- Putting all agreements in writing. This helps to avoid later potential misunderstanding with the understanding that each single agreement is tentative until all are combined into the final package;
- Working out an agenda that is satisfactory to both parties. This includes combining those issues that touch on the same subject and isolating those items peculiar to each opponent;
- Adjourning to study opponent's proposals and preparing for the next meeting.

Your *second meeting* should have at least four purposes. You will want to learn your opponent's overall thinking about his proposals. By questioning him about what he hopes to achieve from this negotiation, you can also get a feel about his priorities and the importance, to him, of each of his agenda items, including his hidden agenda items. When you understand your opponent's fundamental arguments, you will have a basis for more accurately assessing how the meetings will go, and you will be better able to prepare counterarguments and counterproposals. This is the session that should assist you in discovering exactly what is meant by each of the opponent's proposals. Let him know you haven't set your mind for or against any of his proposals. What you are doing is making sure that you really understand what he is proposing before you do take a stand. Question judiciously—clarifying what various words mean both to you and to him. While obtaining this information, you may be able to postpone clarification of your own agenda to the next meeting, thus giving yourself a small edge in the negotiating process.

With the *third session,* you will be reaching for that elusive ideal of *control.* From this point on, you will try to negotiate for your own proposals, whenever they fit in the agreed agenda. Some groundwork may still be necessary to keep your points in discussion, even though most of the second session was used to explore the background of the opponent's proposals. Your approach will be to point out that you have now studied your opponent's proposals and the reasons for putting them forward; that there is merit to some of those proposals which you will address later in the discussion; that there are some proposals you might be able to agree to in principle, but that they are less than acceptable as presented; that your proposals are in keeping with the princples agreed to in the first session, as well as with the generally accepted principles of your specialty society, medical practice, and good business relations; that when serious negotiations begin, your opponent will want to study and understand the reasoning behind your proposals; and, that this will give the opponent time to clarify his thinking about his proposals and their similarity or differences from yours. With that out of the way, adjourn.

While I have outlined three introductory sessions, their content may be condensed into the first session to save time—remember, "quality patient care" is the basis of your arguments whenever possible. One *caveat* should be observed in developing a mutual working agenda. Take care of as many of the non-economic items as you can, before going to the economic ones. Do this for several reasons. It is a truism of negotiating and bargaining that once the money-connected items are agreed upon, one or both parties relax and are ready to go home. They willingly forget non-economic issues, no matter how high they might have been on the priority list. Also, since a major lodestone of administrators in negotiating with hospital-based physicians is directed at cost-containment—and what they choose to designate as too-high earnings—bringing in any talks about money early on will only serve to reinforce their biases. Patient care, administrative difficulties, training, facilities maintenance and modernization, rule and/or regulation updating, deficiencies of hospital administration are some of the issues that can be discussed at length before getting to financial proposals.

As the drama progresses you soon will be in the heart of the real negotiations. To accomplish your goals, a *personal* agenda reflecting your priorities should be carefully prepared before each succeeding meeting. These agendas will include comments or statements and data to supplement your positions, and possible responses to questions the opponent may raise as well as objections and counterproposals to the opponent's earlier arguments. Your comments should be based, for example, upon such background as may be favorable to you from other contracts in your or other hospitals; statistics; specialty practices both local and nationwide; how other hospitals and hospital-based physicians have solved similar mutual problems; and any other credible backup that you can assemble. What you are doing is getting most of the cards on the table so that you may avoid having too many impasse situations. Flexibility and ingenuity should characterize each meeting's preparation. Each of your positions should be sound and defensible, clearly put forward, understandable, fair and reasonable.

A knowledgeable opponent will try to keep you in a defensive position by denigrating your proposals. You must be ready to do the same. Through questions, requests for repetitions, and careful restatements of your opponent's arguments, you can maintain that initiative. Outright opposition is too defensive a tactic—it usually doesn't work to your advantage.

Adopt and Maintain a Personal Negotiating Policy

The objective of any negotiations is a mutually satisfactory agreement. To achieve such an objective, work toward an agreement you feel can be a good working arrangement for you and your opponent. Practical and positive negotiating principles will result in the kind of agreement that you feel you can live with. Avoid doing things that might prevent getting the agreement you want. Basically, you should:

- **Start with, and maintain, a positive negotiating deportment.** For example, at the first meeting you might make a statement something like this, "We are both here with the interests of our patients as prime concern. Let's work toward what is fair and best for them, and the results will surely benefit us." Begin by making it impossible for your opponent to disagree with you. If you sit down with the attitude that "I won't agree to anything until you make me," you will be sure to generate forces that will be to your disadvantage.
- **Recognize that your opponent's position is not always entirely his own.** He represents a board of directors or the senior administrator who gave him a set of goals and he has to satisfy some of those or lose his job.
- **Realize that you may have to persuade your opponent to change the opinions he brought to the table.** Let him know that you recognize the sincerity of his beliefs, but that in order for you to perform proficiently in the hospital, together you will have to work out another solution that is mutually satisfactory and beneficial.
- **Keep in mind the realization that what is perfectly understandable to you as a physician may be neither understandable nor logical to a balance-sheet-oriented administrator.** You will approach certain issues with similar mental blocks. You might find that you have to spend some of your negotiating time broadening your opponent's horizons and understanding. When either basic differences or lack of understanding intrude into a discussion, you can keep the meeting

from degenerating into a brouhaha of name-calling or worse by moving to another subject with something like "We could undoubtedly disagree over this problem for the rest of this session without converting either of us, so let's agree to disagree for the moment and move on to item X. We're here to negotiate an agreement, so let's talk about the things we have a chance of settling and think about our positions after we adjourn."

- **Examine and restate your opponent's proposal or counterproposal—question and listen—for areas where you can both agree, if only in principle.** Differences are often not more than what words have come to mean to people. If you can find the similarities of meaning between you, agreement usually follows.
- **Emphasize the differences if you are on a subject where you do not want to agree.** Agreement becomes impossible as long as the *differences* continue to be the basis of discussion. Logic, as well as an emphasis on the real meaning of the words being used, can be utilized to create understanding. And repetition, of logic and other facets of your position, can work for you in presenting your positive negotiating attitude.
- **Maintain a cordial atmosphere.** Newton's first law of physics applies to the negotiation process. You get, in return, what you give. Misrepresentations beget misrepresentations. Name-calling, verbal abuse, indulgence in personality derogation, and shouting will be returned to the sender. Sincerity, fairness, callness, and credibility also will be returned to the sender resulting in more productive negotiations.
- **Keep the negotiations moving along.** When discussions start to drag, a number of things can be done to get them moving again. Pass on to another subject as was suggested earlier. If the dragging is coming from someone bringing in tangential subjects or unrelated items, bring the discussion back to the topic at hand with "What you are saying is interesting, but it doesn't seem to be helping us get any closer to solving the problem we were discussing. We're here to get a workable agreement. Why not spend our time on those things we are both concerned with and save our efforts for discussing those items that will work to both our and our patients' advantage. That way we can save time and effort by leaving out those subjects that keep us from our goals."

- **Personalize progress and depersonalize obstructive attitudes.** When the administrator or his associate directs movement that is constructive, sound, and furthers your cause, show your appreciation and agreement. Should their action be off-base, malicious, witless, or ridiculous, and some response is called for to keep the discussion to the subject, point out that the conversation—not the person—is pursuing an unsound tack or that the statement is inaccurate. Don't imply that the person making the statement is personally responsible for it.
- **Put the burden of proof on your opponent.** Question him as to why the change or the point he is trying to make is fair to both sides, workable, and suitable. No agreement should be made until he proves his point to your satisfaction. If his position has merit and substance, you must proceed accordingly. If, however, there is no merit or substance to the proposal, trying to prove his point will indicate bases for non-agreement. Substantiating an invalid argument will help him convince himself that he was on unsound ground to begin with.
- **Stay away from questions that can be answered with a simple yes or no.** You want the answers to your questions in the form of statements. Questions developed around a *who, what, where, when, why,* and *how* will be helpful in pushing discussion to either agreement or dropping the subject. The answers to these questions will be useful if you have to summarize an opponent's position when it contradicts his original stand.

6
YOUR ROLE AS NEGOTIATOR

Very learned people are easy to deceive because, although they are versed in abstruse matters, they lack the more necessary knowledge of everyday affairs.

Baltasar Gracian, S. J. (circa 1720)

Those who have spent time negotiating successfully will tell you that provoking your opponent and threatening his self-respect, status, or integrity is likely to create intangible issues that may become more important than the specific issues about which the negotiations are being conducted. When intangible issues come to the fore either because of excessive demands or obstructive behavior, an opponent may feel victimized and respond in a retaliatory manner. Or, he may do his best to restore some semblance to the meetings. Whether one handles such a situation in the manner of a Machiavelli: "If an injury has to be done to a man it should be so severe that his vengence should not be feared," or of Pollyanna: "Everything will be all right if we look on the bright side" becomes a matter of personal attitude. I prefer the "don't get mad, get even" approach. But in getting even, do it in a way that doesn't make a bitter enemy of your opponent.

Some may look upon negotiations as a game rather than a means or process. What may lead to such a conclusion is the emphasis upon either gamesmanship play or the tactics promoted by writers using titles like *Power Negotiating, Getting Yours,* etc. But negotiating is not a game. In the early stages, the development will appear to be nothing but shadow-boxing "I want . . ." ". . . you can't be serious . ." ". . . and my reasons are . . " "I don't understand your logic. Please tell me . . ." and so on.

Hospital administrators, along with their lawyers, have become adept at shaping a superior and winning facade for the professionals using their facilities. Physicians can learn from the one-upmanship that is continually practiced. The gambits and ploys that they utilize, as well as some of the countermeasures are described below. A physician with average negotiating ability and the willingness to exercise some *chutzpah* can protect himself in the clinches.

Using Deadlines

Time can be an important component of negotiating strategy. How your opponent makes use of your time can play into his hands. In most negotiating situations, the pressure of either real or assumed deadlines has a tendency to make opponents more flexible as negotiations move along. The lack of progress as time passes somehow manages to cause one's expectations to decline. Although considerable time can be taken up with the discussions and explanations of objectives, enough time must be reserved to allow for the nitty-gritty that will achieve that win/win result. As the parties discuss their problems, they come to the realization that the totality of the goals that they brought to the table may be out of reach for this negotiation. On the other hand, the discussions may have brought out more areas of common ground so that they both become more willing to compromise. Negotiations demand a willingness to compromise goals that are either unattainable or out of line. If there is an attitude of unrest among hospital staff it might be best to work for a short negotiation and a quick settlement so that you may extract major concessions before your opponent has time to solve his morale problem. However, if major issues have to be resolved, you should not rush. One last caveat on time—stop when you have the best solution to your problem. If you oversell or overstroke your opponent, you may lose much of what you have gained.

The tactics available to negotiators are as numerous and as varied as are the people who use them. There are two basic types: those concerned with minimizing conflict, and those that assist in getting your points across. The Pollyanna approach or Conflict Reducing, works from two basic principles: disclosing your priorities and presenting your goals in such a manner that it causes your opponent minimal obvious surrender of his positions. Machiavellian tactics are the pressure tools you can use to accomplish and improve your negotiating situations.

As with any interpersonal relationship, it is important to maintain control of the situation as it progresses. If you are well prepared and can somehow control the timing and concentration of the discussions, you will maintain your expectations. Your confidence will affect your opponent, carrying him along with you. Convince your opponent that you are serious about this negotiation and that you are there to negotiate sincerely, credibly and certainly in good faith. By letting him know that you have prepared for these discussions and are probably better informed about the subject matter than he (not by bragging, but by performance) he may be more likely to try to meet you better than half way. After all, negotiation is a form of salesmanship, and the secret of successful salespeople is making the sale valuable to both parties. The person who does best in most negotiations is one who negotiates low-key, but is not bored or lackadaisical. The trick is to be low-key, but insistent and persistent. Don't overdo the tactical stratagem. One properly chosen tactic will be more valuable to you than will many poorly selected tactics. Be aware of your opponent's reaction to a tactic before pursuing an expected result. Don't be afraid to let the issues shape the tenor of a negotiations, keeping in mind that you are there to work with your opponent to get the best deal you can make.

Back to Pollyanna or Machiavelli.

The Pollyanna Approach

If you go into a negotiation with the idea of avoiding or minimizing the possibilities of conflict and disharmony, you will probably put your objectives on the table in order of their priorities, most important first. Then you make it known that you do not intend to spend too much time negotiating minor issues until the important items have been taken care of. This approach is alright if your opponent is willing to take the same one that you are, and if the negotiation is about limited objectives. If, however, a number of difficult problems must be resolved, you should present your issues in something other than priority order. That order should be based upon how you visualize the potential linkages with concession-influencing arguments that may come up during the discussions. You may find it advisable to direct the early talks around those positive components in your opponent's favor, especially if these are your secondary goals. Opponents often agree on some secondary proposals to get negotiations moving. Some objectives that may be essential to you but not so obvious to your opponent can be brought into the discussion while he is conceding secondary or nonessential objectives. Unless he is insisting on compensating concessions in these early stages, he puts you into a reasonably good position to avoid having to make balancing concessions.

For example, you are negotiating an exclusive service agreement with your hospital. Your group is willing to provide twenty-four hour coverage in your specialty, but because of the estimated potential need for your services and the estimated income available, it would not be financially prudent to fully staff the group for onsite availability. By directing the discussion to the hospital's needs and reasons for twenty-four hour *availability,* you propose that, since the need for your specialty's service are usually called for and required within a certain time frame, you will guarantee service within _____ minutes of a call to either a group telephone number or the scheduled physician. Of course, any such agreement should be written as clearly as possible. Be careful with early concessions. Making them too early and too easily may lead your opponent to think that he has a patsy for an opponent. Once started on a pattern of minor, but easy-to-make one-sided concessions, it is difficult to become tough and demanding when negotiations get more serious. Remember that negotiating is a search for common ground. If, during the early stages of negotiation, an agreement on an opponent's goal or yours—no matter how important or minor an objective it may be—seems imminent, postpone settlement until both parties may be better prepared to finalize several issues.

The other aspect of the pollyanna approach is to structure your goals so that an opponent will find that he can accept them with minimal apparent sacrifice of his position. Too often, opponents resist making concessions because they feel that by doing so they will be put in a position that causes them to lose face or to be embarrassed. Rather than expecting your opponent to accept a radical change in his objectives, develop his potential acceptance by being flexible and inventive in pursuing and restating your goals. By being perceptive, and introducing nonmaterial or nonfinancial benefits—either real or imaginative, so that the apparent cost to him is minor, you will improve your chances that he will compromise or concede a point.

The Machiavelli Approach

What follows are descriptions of ploys that can be used to enhance the acceptability of one's position or appeal to an opponent's need to settle.

They can be used to inhibit or deter an opponent from taking or continuing an undesirable position, or to maximize one's own negotiating stance. Consensus is what we are seeking, and if the proper use of these tactics—or variations thereof—will assist you in instilling either uncertainty, apprehension, expectation, or greed into an opponent's posture at the table, their use can be justified. However, at times, certain tactics, even when correctly used, will not work because of the skill or experience level of the other person. What can be realistically expected from your knowledge and use of tactics as described will be the possibility of an edge in carrying on the negotiations dialogue. If they do not prove productive, or if they are tried on you, you will be aware of the reasons and you will be able to defend yourself.

Tactics fall into at least four general categories. They can be: diversionary; evaluative or personalized; defensive or inhibiting; and cooperative or reassuring. As we go along you will see that certain tactics may be used in several of these categories interchangeably. What you have here is a buffet of ploys. And, as with any buffet, you will have to taste or experiment, testing them in various negotiations to learn which work best for you and with which you are most comfortable. How you use them will be important. One successful tactic is better than four or five inappropriate ones. Be comfortable with what you are trying. If it works, fine. If it doesn't, try again. Don't fret, you have the whole buffet to choose from. One caveat. Don't become so enamoured of a few tactics that you use and reuse them repeatedly in successive negotiations without variation. Your opponent will quickly learn what to expect, and will lead you into a lose/win result. Since we have been preaching win/win results for the negotiating process, let us first look at cooperative and reassuring tactics.

Concede, Convert and Proceed

When an opponent sets out certain conditions that he has to have to make a deal worthy of serious consideration, consider them. As long as these conditions, in total or in large part do not destroy your negotiating expectations, you have little to lose by going along. An administrator negotiating an exclusive agreement with a hospital-based physician may require certain non-financial duties—teaching, administration, report writing, supervision, or direction. How will these duties impinge upon your ability to provide the medical services needed? If these requests are common to your specialty, accede. By going along, you are building your credibility, setting bases for requiring later concessions, and designing his investment in the ultimate settlement. However, in going along, begin with a tentative yes. Be ready to question for details—including when, what, how, where, and with whom. Similarly, you may be able to buy your opponent's objections to some of your proposals. Again, as long as these objections do not restrict your ability to provide your services, go along carefully. The objections may be real or contrived. If they are real, they should be cleared up. If, however, after you have gone along, your opponent is still less-than-eager to move to settlement, you have at least pushed the contrived issues out of the way (and, at an appropriate time, may find occasion to gently renege, with "new" reasons for changing your agreement). You now should smoke out the underlying problems. Often in negotiations an opponent is reluctant to disclose a problem or is emotionally unable to agree to your solution. By infiltrating his facade you bring out the real problem, and have an opportunity to work out a solution. Situations where an opponent is acting as someone's agent, with definite limits to what he is able to agree will develop a lot of objections. At such times it will be best to restrict your bargaining points until your opponent either gets his authority extended, or someone who can make an agreement that will stick comes into the negotiation.

Problem Solving

When both parties come to the table intending to work out an agreement, but don't seem to be able to get together on the particulars of how, the opportunity for problem-solving is auspicious. Both sides have objectives with which the other has become knowledgeable, and both want to settle. If both parties work together to develop alternative approaches to work around a problem, they both stand to gain, even though neither gets everything he came to the table for. By getting your opponent to work with you in formulating a solution on the basis of the facts both have brought forth, you get him committed to a reasonably satisfactory alternative to which he contributed. For example, most contracts and agreements being presented to hospital-based physicians omit any reference to due-process for the physicians while reserving the right to terminate the contract or agreement within a limited period for any or no reason. Usually the sections assigned to such "managerial rights" are tightly worded and placed at the tail-end of the write-up after all the "important issues" are taken care of. They are often overlooked. This creates a need for problem solving. The physician must ask questions and offer alternatives.

The primary motive for problem solving is to get away from the obstructions that too often result from the personalized viewpoints of the negotiators. Both sides come to the table with strong opinions and developing alternatives is not an easy task. Nitpicking proposals for new approaches before discussing the options prematurely, limits your ability to negotiate creatively. Finally, any problems requiring ingenuity and tact should not be directed back to the negotiator as his problem alone—if all problems are treated as expressions of mutual interest, each is then in a position to become part of the solution. Create options first, find a way to enlarge the available boundaries of the subject under discussion, then evaluate the options and their potential benefits to both parties. Define the problem, discuss the symptoms and causes of the problem, and select the solution that seems best for both parties.

Objectivity, Fairness, Reasonableness, and Playing Devil's Advocate

No matter how much we advocate the development of a win/win attitude, particularly in continuing relationships, we have to admit that there will be conflicting interests at work. Too often the resolution of these conflicts ends up in horse-trading that only postpones the ultimate breakdown of that relationship. What is needed is for both parties to stand away from their ego-involvement and to work together for an objective solution based upon each side establishing fair and reasonable standards. With objectivity, they can mutually work to a solution that benefits both while leaving their psyches intact.

For example, a hospital-based physician group, renegotiating a multiyear exclusive service agreement, included in its proposals a need for a free-standing commerical laboratory in the community. The hospital insisted that if the group ran the laboratory, there would be a serious conflict of interest. The spokesman for the group, explaining that the group had no desire or intent to divert any laboratory work presently being done in the hospital, pointed out that present budgets make no provision for new equipment or updating equipment in use, and that other hospitals within the drawing area were in a similar situation. What the group was proposing would be a service to the community and the hospital. Objectively, what alternatives could the hospital propose?

Fairness, reasonableness, good faith, and objectivity—all are being stressed from your opponent's point of view. Each of you at the table is trying to maximize his negotiating results. If you stand steady on certain issues, fair to you, does that mean you are being unreasonable? Such accusations are usually tactical appeals.

The devil's advocate approach can be used to further involve an opponent in a cooperative effort to a problem solution. ''What if . . . .'' and ''had you thought about . . . . .?'' sort of questions serve to pique an occasionally recalcitrant opponent's interest enough to at least raise objections. With the back and forth discussion of alternatives, the negotiations can be kept moving toward satisfactory solutions.

Now, for the tactics of diversion. A negotiator may attempt to get you involved in confusing side issues that will eventually put you in the ''gotta get it settled before it's too late'' attitude. Or, if you are making a solid, straightforward presentation, he'll interrupt you—anything to keep you from accomplishing an objective that he isn't ready or willing to make concessions on. Recognize these as diversions; treat them as such; and continue with your presentation. Conversational leadings such as ''Frankly, I . . . .,'' ''By the way, have you . . . .,'' ''Incidentally . . .,'' ''Before we get too far into . . .,'' ''Yes, but . . .,'' may be diversions. In negotiations, as with any drama, it takes a lot of character development and situation development before the action peaks and the play works to its conclusion. The ''Pareto principle'' is a generalization that states 80 percent of the ''action'' in any confrontation takes place in the last 20 percent or less of the time available to the parties. This is when the pressure is placed on the party that has perhaps dawdled too long and too often over non-essentials, forcing the party into premature decisions or overgenerous concessions.

Deadlines, Delays, and Speedups

Some deadlines are rigid as in contract endings or application submissions. Others are unilaterally or self-imposed and leave room for negotiating. Establishing or threatening to set a deadline applies pressure to both parties to overcome the inertia of inconclusive negotiating and to move on to more productive bargaining. Pacing oneself toward a deadline results in productive solutions. Allowing an opponent to stampede one into a quick settlement will usually result in an unfavorable solution. If a deadline is real, work toward it. If it is a ploy, work toward it but not under the pressure of *having* to finish within the allotted time. And, in most cases, whether real or a ploy, *if* progress is being made, deadlines can be extended by mutual agreement for specific limited times. One important note about deadline negotiating—*if you've been at it for some hours and you're tired and edgy, adjourn the meeting or caucus to "recharge" your energies.* Decisions made under the pressures of deadlines that could have been adjusted have a tendency to be poor ones. It's better to be sure of what you are doing than to have to live with something neither party is happy with. If you need time to clarify or solidify the particulars of a final agreement with an imminent deadline, don't forget *patient care.*

Using delay tactics can be helpful when, after several sessions of exchanging information and clearing the air, you want to find out how anxious your opponent is to agree on an issue. Foot dragging, because of patient requirements or the need for attendance at a CME (continuing medical education) session, preferably out of town, might offer your opponent an incentive to settle the issue now. Recognize a delay tactic for a pressure if it is tried on you—and calmly set the date for the next meeting, noting some objectives you want on that upcoming agenda.

If negotiations have been characterized by a lot of talk but limited progress, some form of speedup may be in order. Push for clear and positive answers to your questions, and propose settlements that they have to refuse. Keep after them for alternatives, offering some of your own, with "if's" and "maybe's" while politely demanding answers. However, unless you are willing to move to another hospital, or have been recruited to possibly move, speedup tactics have a way of backfiring, so be careful.

Sidetracking, Red Herrings, and Authority Limits

Sidetracking can be the ultimate Machiavellian technique. Say that you are having a difficult time with a very tough administrator. There is no "give", only an attitude of "gimme." Logic, facts, stroking, nothing works to get him into a negotiating stance. You may be able to have him sidetracked by using another ploy, the end run. If you know where his authority comes from, or know someone who does, get the message to that authority about how well their negotiator is doing—holding to his objectives, not giving a centimeter, tough and rude and acting as though the hospital is his, how the physician morale is down because of his no-concession attitude. If the ploy works, you have set up a delay that should give you an opportunity to promote the objectives that were being ignored.

If this tactic is not to your taste, try to make that tough opponent look, and feel, unreasonable. Because he has put you in a position of giving concessions on an "or else" basis while granting nothing in return, the approach might be "Look, we're as interested in getting an agreement as you are, and we've been doing all the giving without any getting. From here on in it's your turn or we'll have to pass the word around that you're not interested in maintaining a cooperative organization.'' Or, ''Your attitude of refusing to substantiate your position is unreasonable and not in keeping with the leadership aura that you promote. We need the backup to understand where you're coming from in this discussion, so either tell us or get someone in here who can.'' Should you find yourself on the receiving end of such ploys, keep your cool and explain that your firm stand is for the benefit and best interests of both parties. Or, you might want to act defensive saying, ''Good heavens, do I have to go over the whole thing, again? Why can't you take my word that that's the way it will work or show me why it won't?''

Red herrings, straw men, waving the yellow flag—are all names for diversionary tactics that can be used to sidetrack the opponent. The red herring may be be an outright lie or misrepresentation that shifts the blame for lack of negotiating progress to the other side, by introducing what appears to be a logical and plausible argument that the opponent will have trouble ignoring. A red herring is, by nature, vague and indefinite and is based on faceless and nondiscoverable sources. Since a red herring is thrown into the discussion as a diversion, putting the burden either directly or indirectly on you, denials, no matter how justified or sincere, only serve to embroil you in a no-win situation. The best way to protect yourself against red herrings that are thrown at you is to ignore them, change the subject of the discussion, or diligently question for the source of the statements. The best counter of the three mentioned above is to ignore the ploy—bring the opponent back to the subject that was being discussed or bring up a new one.

Authority limits, used sparingly, can be a valuable tactic. A negotiator who is representing his partnership or group is not an autonomous person. He may have negotiating freedom, but when faced with concessions that are difficult, he can always tell his opponent that a particular concession is beyond his authority. This is a tactic often used by hospital administrators. You are led to assume that the higher authority or the other members of the group have a much tougher attitude than the negotiator, and are more likely to turn down whatever it is that the current negotiator might be willing to agree to. So, rather than disturb the momentum and lose the opportunity for a reasonable gain, you—or he—go along with lesser gains. If you are convinced that your opponent is playing games with his approved limits, you can either insist upon negotiating only with the person who does have final authority or demand that the present opponent not return to the table until he has authority to work within a larger potential range for settlement. The higher powers that you refer to while negotiating—"What you are saying sounds pretty good to me, but I'd better see what my boss/partner/board thinks before I say yes. . ."—may not exist, but your opponent doesn't have to know that. It is important to sound out your opponent and see if he has the final authority. Is he able to make deals and commit his organization, or is he someone sent to the table to absorb your information, use up your valuable time, and finally tell you that he hasn't the authority to settle? The bureaucratic maze can be effective in wearing you down and forcing additional concessions out of you as you struggle to settle with the different levels of authority. Until you have determined your opponent's authority limits, make your concessions difficult or tentative and insist upon getting a *quid pro quo* for each. Remember, if you bare your soul at the early negotiating stages, you will have no leverage when the more powerful opponent comes to the table.

One of the major aims in any win/win negotiation is to achieve a settlement that places your opponent at, or a little below his bottom line. You want to move the opponent to settle to your advantage. By using defensive tactics, you can inhibit the expectations that he brought to the table. You'll need these tactics when your opponent is doing better than you are, when his expectations are too high or unreasonable, and when you need to learn more about him in order to negotiate intelligently. Your credibility will be at stake in using some of these tactics. You do not want to be seen as trying to bluff or threaten. Credibility evolves from consistency, patience and persistence, with the backup of good preparation. One of the means by which you can utilize your credibility to increase your potential for success is to present multiple choice options so that refusal of all becomes difficult. If you can present a series of reasonable and comparable alternatives, you are offering them more ways to say yes. For example, you propose 24-hour availability and/or consultative management service for the hospital's outpatient service locations and/or some additional minor goal that the hospital may want, and something that is important to your objectives as possibilities. More options, singly or in combination, will increase the yes potential. And, if you can include an alternative that can only require a definite no, you have tossed in a red herring that increases the chances of a yes to something you want. "Which of these is most agreeable to you . . .?" Any time you can offer more than one option you increase your chances of developing a yes.

A variation of the multiple choice proposition is to develop your objectives, where possible, as a series of smaller objectives. What you try for is to work your opponent into agreeing to a number of minor proposals, leading to a climax that almost precludes a no. But the tactic works both ways. If it's thrown at you and you see it developing, stall. Put it aside for study or to discuss with your party, and change the topic of discussion.

Any time you are proposing multiple alternatives to push for a yes, you should be thinking of the possible nonfinancial or ego costs for your opponent that might be involved in his conceding or agreeing. Reducing or eliminating any such apparent cost will increase the potential for consessions or agreement. Flexibility and imagination, getting out of the ruts into which too many of us allow ourselves to travel, will increase your chances for better than average success.

Black Hat, White Hat, Mincing, Linkage

Call it by any of a number of names—''black hat-white hat'', ''bad guy-good guy'', this is strictly a role-playing act by members of the opponent's team. The black hat/bad guy is the difficult, vituperative, unreasonable negotiator who seeks to coerce you and your associates into acquiesence. During a break or caucus, a white hat/good guy pulls you aside and suggests unhappiness with his team member's attitude and proposes to work within his team for a more moderate alternative—usually a more reasonable proposal that his team is really after—to get your confidence. With that confidence, he can more easily probe for your bottom lines and other truths that were previously held back. What you are being dealt is an obvious but seemingly subliminal swap of courtesy and humanity for negotiating stress relief. If the tactic is tried on you, don't pay any attention to the perpetrators. Don't get upset by the bad guy's intransigence. Disregard his histrionics and concentrate on the proposals and alternatives of his alter ego. And, if the bad guy continues his noisy and threatening way, propose to your good guy that his partner change his approach, leave the room until he calms down, or you will recess the meeting to another time. As for the good guy, he isn't there to pass out goodies for your benefit; he is inviting you to accept something less than you want or need, but you don't have to jump. Let him know that you expect him to do better. Or, if you are the kind of person who every once-in-a-while like to puncture balloons, look the good guy in the eye, smile, and tell him ''Say, your buddy sure does play at wearing his black hat very well.''

Mincing, too, goes by a number of names—salami tactic, nibbling, dessert-on-the-house—and is useful in a number of ways. You can mince both up and down. Mincing up consists primarily of creating a series of positive responses to minimal concessions or agreements by stroking an opponent. Each small "yes" builds upon the last ones without revealing the final proposal—the objective. What you are doing—and this is a tactic not to be overused, but when used, must be well-planned—is repeatedly getting a foot in the door, or as Edward Bennett Williams describes the tactic: "You peel the onion layer by layer. You don't begin by stabbing for the heart."

Mincing down comes into play at a point when the negotiations are at the final agreement. At that moment one of the parties comes up with a request for a "little sweetener" to make the deal more palatable for his backers. Too often, the object of that request, either feeling good about the deal he already has or afraid that by turning down the sweetener he will lose his deal, agrees. This tactic is also tried after the parties have agreed upon the total results of their negotiations with the ploy that one of the parties coming back to the table claiming that his principals are willing to settle, *but* certain items require slight revision (in their favor, of course) or expansion. Credibility is at stake here. Once the deal has been made, stick to it! And make your opponent live up to his committments! While you both have an investment of time, effort and potential goodies that you don't want to lose because of some small "gimmees," in cases of mincing going beyond that which you agreed to in good faith. The other party will quickly withdraw if the proposal is quickly and firmly refused—after all, he wants the deal to hold up too. So, if this tactic is tried on you, refuse with amazement, with indignation, and with "You've got to be kidding!"

Through linkage you work with what may best be described as conditional arrangements. They are "I can probably see giving you that point, *if* . . .", or "Before we get too involved with these details we have to settle the problem of . . ." Linked issues should be settled as close to the same time as possible. They are an excellent way to bring your important objectives to the table in a way that makes it difficult for an opponent to avoid and to keep negotiating on a *quid pro quo* basis.

Working Together

Personalizing the negotiating relationship can be pursued in several ways. When one is interested in developing or maintaining a good working relationship, care must be taken not to offend the opponent. When one does not care about the relationship, a variety of adversarial tactics may be put to use. A good working relationship promotes open dialogue, allows the parties to introduce off-the-record "trial balloons" into the conversation for frank and private solution explorations, and, usually, fosters the expectation of a good post-negotiation relationship. With a good personal relationship, credibility and trust have been established over time by the parties' punctual completion of their negotiated commitments to the point where, *contrary to a basic premise advocated by this negotiator to always get the agreement in writing and initialed,* the parties work on handshakes and understanding. One thing to think about in handshake situations: you both represent other opposing, parties. Changes take place. When a crunch comes, will you both be there to settle on the basis of your friendship and understanding? Will different people accept your word? Don't depend on it—memo your agreement for posterity.

Where there has not been a long-term relationship but there is a chance that a personal relationship could develop you should do an in-depth research job on your opponent. Learn all you can about the things that annoy the other party, about his idiosyncracies both at work and at the negotiating table, and check them out as the negotiations proceed. For the inexperienced physician-negotiator who may be the object of being personalized by a more experienced hospital representative, be careful and, perhaps, a bit cynical. Personalization can blunt one's alertness by developing an unfounded confidence in the relationship. Because an experienced negotiator is always probing and reaching for settlement whether at the table or at a social situation where there is a tendency to relax, you must keep up your guard if you feel you are being personalized.

Ethics

Having been trained at considerable length to be ethical in their medical practice, physicians occasionally question whether the realities of negotiating are ethical. Perhaps the reason for raising the issue is basic concern with the limits you may or may not observe in promoting your cause. Understandably, you will want to maintain your credibility, arrive at a win/win solution, and be "fair." All these have merit of course, but the *impression* of fairness and ethicality that one projects as part of his aura of credibility is extremely important. And, it will usually follow that in creating this impression, the pragmatic result will be "working" ethics. However, at all times the physician-negotiator should be aware that his opponents probably have no qualms about leading him down a primrose path with misleading statements, exaggeration, and yes, even on occasion, lies in order to advance their position. How a negotiator answers ethical questions is a personal decision. As a general guide, a negotiator should practice being "ethical" until, because of his opponent's conduct, he sees his own ethical stance becoming a burden that precludes a favorable outcome to the negotiation. As a negotiator, you do not have to be a rogue to be successful, but you must recognize unethical behavior and be prepared to fight fire with fire or have some other effective means to counter it.

A personal code, beyond which one would be seriously uncomfortable in proceeding, is indispensable to the question of ethical practice. Your code should involve three considerations: the possible deleterious effect upon the long-term relationship; the possible exposure to unfavorable career-related disciplinary or other action; and the possible effect of such action upon one's reputation or one's credibility both as a person and as a negotiator. Two basic principles bind these together: (1) a promise made is a promise to be kept; and (2) don't promise something you can't deliver.

If you are not concerned with developing or maintaining a long-term relationship with your opponent, you can use tactics that are intended to make him uncomfortable. These include such tactics as making him appear unreasonable, making personal attacks on the opponent's character and credibility (not too difficult with many administrators who often contradict themselves by trying to please everybody at the same time), expressing boredom with the opponent's proposals, emphasizing your vulnerable position, and making the opponent appear to be the problem at the table. Your concern is to put him on the defensive. But be careful—he can do the same thing to you, using the media and bureaucratic attacks on the profession to support his charges. At that point you can either ignore his charges, or reply that it is ridiculous to judge an entire profession on distorted accounts of isolated incidents.

As with Machiavelli, any or all of these and other tactics you will learn to use, should reinforce your position at the negotiating table. Please, divest yourself—doctor—of any illusions of indispensability when you are negotiating for yourself or for a group. There is nothing wrong with using any ploy to convince an opponent of indispensability; just don't begin to believe it yourself, because indispensable people are expendable—especially in today's hospital survival situations. Mutual interests, of which we have written earlier, will help to personalize your relations with an opponent. Develop them, use them, and find ways to convert your problems into *our* problems. Gratitude is an ephemeral quality in negotiations and hospital management. The bottom line has no morals, and professional management few loyalties. Hospital management, as with any business, works for its own interests and not by sentiment. But—don't forget—they need you, no matter how they describe, design, and delimit both their and your autonomy.

The following list contains examples of several different tactics and attitudes which you may employ as you negotiate. Become familiar with these tactics so that you'll recognize them when your opponent uses them.

Fraternity

Exploiting an existing fraternal association can be an effective negotiating strategy. The negotiator has a choice of several sibling-like attitudes to choose from when using this strategy, including: Brothers-on-a-par: equal in power, status and need; Senior brother: age has responsibilities to be kind; Baby brother: last in needs help; and Prodigal brother: make up for lost time.

However, don't depend too much on the expected goodnesses of assumed fraternalism. "Help me" can, and often does, get one help in ways that harm rather than help.

Casting Stones

Guilt-peddling is often a matter of perspective. Pursuit of your objectives does not imply that you are trying to take advantage of an opponent with whom you have had a good relationship. However, he may try to make you feel guilty with remarks like:

> "After all that we've worked on so well together, you do this to me?"? or
> "Why are you asking for so much more from me than from all the other staff doctors? You don't hear them demanding more than their due."; or
> "I thought that we understood each other better than that."; etc.

If you are negotiating above board and feel comfortable pursuing your goals, why feel guilty?

Flattery and Charm

Sycophancy, or playing to your ego, can be one of the more insidious tactics used to exploit a personal relationship. Being told what an excellent physician you are, how esteemed you are in the medical and consumer communities, that you are worth more than you are asking, *but* your demands can't be met, is a good example of this tactic. Be sure that the soft soap and the ego-stroking do not interfere with your bargaining effort.

Who's Buying/Who's Selling

Often an opponent will take the offensive with a salvo of questions and statements that are directed to one end—is this the proper position for you? The answer that should come to your mind is—who should be selling whom here? This issue becomes one of where the need lies. Yes, you have had an exclusive agreement with the hospital for a long time, and you fear a move to another medical staff, but why, after all this time should they seek change? The problem is to detour this attempt to put you on the defensive by getting your opponent to convince you why you should continue making your services available to his hospital staff. Facts, not presumptive arrogance, should convey the idea that he needs you at least as much as you need him. There's nothing wrong with a little guilt-peddling in a situation such as this.

When You're Right, You're Right

There will be times when an opponent will repeat false or half-true statements about you or something you are supposed to have done. This is the time to get mad, to rant and rave, to threaten to go over your opponent's head, and to start backing out of all earlier committments and concessions. By making manifest how seriously you take these apparent slurs on your character and reputation, you discourage them from pursuing this line of attack.

Authority, Legitimacy, Expertise

I often have occasion to recall a poster on a machine-shop wall that read: "When all else fails, read the instructions." Any number of authority-conscious administrators will pull rank and apparent knowledge to make you back off a negotiating goal. In your specialty, you are the "expert." Status, reputation, credibility all combine to give you an element of negotiating power that an opponent may be trying to denigrate. You can tactfully remind your opponent of those elements within the framework of the current situation, and where possible effectuate your expertise with medical gobbledegook that has to be explained—but not too often.

Precedents

The precedent-setting character of concession-making during negotiations and incident-settling during the life of an agreement are legitimate concerns. Often, because of the perceived potential effect of a precedential act, an opponent will avoid approaching an agreement. When you are up against such precedent fear, be understanding and work toward an alternative solution that won't threaten the bogey of precedent in his mind. One-time concession settlements, agreed to as "non-precedential" are seldom such. Invariably, one or the other party finds an excuse at later negotiations to refer to "that settlement we made on ______" as the precedent for pushing for a current concession. In such cases, all you can do is point out the "non-precedent" agreement that was the basis for the previous agreement, and move on to alternatives or another subject—unless the combination of previous and/or potential concessions towards your goals for this negotiation appears to be advantageous.

Finally, precedent-pointing is the perennial fallback of bureaucrats and institutional people. "That's the way it's done," or "That's the policy," or "The regulations say ______". Ask to see the rule, regulation, or law. If it is actually in print, was it published in some official source? Quite often you will find interoffice memos or interpretations that protect the bureaucrats. Ignore these. Go back to the published, printed rule, regulation, or law, and work from that. Offer alternative goal-concession arrangements as a means to break through the bureaucratic barrier. You will often find that while a bureaucrat retreats to the cocoon of his rules and regulations, a strain of rebellion can be brought out by suggesting a way to beat those bindings.

By now you have the idea that quite a number of tactical maneuvers and ploys are available. Obviously only a few have been covered here. To detail them in total in their many variations would require a *Kama Sutra* of tactics. There is no magic formula for negotiating success; innumerable options are open to you. How you apply tactics to effectuate your basic negotiating strategy for the meetings with an opponent should have one fundamental purpose; to achieve a win/win solution to current problems by offering the opponent an elevated satisfaction level while chopping away at his aspirations. Just remember that you should not become so enamoured of certain tactics that they become your permanent weapons, leaving you open to being typecast and taken. Be *flexible* and *comfortable* as you negotiate, and you'll find the process more enjoyable and beneficial.

7
REFINING YOUR SKILLS

Man was given the gift of speech in order that he might disguise his thoughts.
Charles Maurice de Talleyrand

By now it should be clear that negotiating is a less than precise art. It could, perhaps, be likened to the study and practice of law—much more clinical than precise when it is applied, and seldom concrete. One learns the ground rules, and, with dismay, finds that no factor is a constant, no rule inviolate. However, with planning, research, and an empathy for flexibility, one can create an image and develop the ability to converse and, perhaps, convert one's opponent.

Conversation has to be a two-way street. Pacing one's silences, one's listening, keeps the street open and traffic moving. The more the traffic moves, the more opportunities to increase knowledge of one's opponent—why he is your opponent, what he will concede to get as much of whatever it is that he really wants and needs. You will learn how flexible he is in understanding your goals, whether his apparent obstinacy is subjective or pressed upon him by others. Listening, with understanding—hearing with thoughtful attention rather than merely perceiving the sounds coming from across the table—is the difference between success and mediocrity in negotiating.

How a negotiator presents the case can make the difference between having an opponent listen and understand what is being suggested and why, or having the opponent just sit there hearing what is being said while waiting to have a say. From the beginning, the negotiator must learn, and consciously practice, language that avoids misunderstanding. Too often, professionals, entranced with and embalmed in their professional jargon, talk in what sounds to an uninitiated listener like "blah blah blah." English has many words that sound the same, but mean different things. If, as one talks, one sees questions, or blank looks, on the face of that person sitting opposite, stop talking. Think about what has been said. At such times—and there can be several in the course of a meeting—it becomes advisable to ask whether there is any question about what has been said. It is even better, after stopping, to take a few moments to explain, or define the words that you have been using. "' _____ ', for me, means ' _____ _____ _____,'" or, "This means ' _____ ' for me, how do you understand (or, what does it mean to you?)." By the same token, if there is any question in your mind about what your opponent is saying, ask at the earliest possible moment—without interrupting: "Do you mean ' _____ _____ _____?'" or restate the thought in your own words. Clarity and understanding will make any negotiation successful in finding that middle ground that both seek.

Listeners face a variety of potential misunderstandings when what they hear appears conditional. If several alternatives are to be placed on the table think such a presentation through before blurting it out. Your preparation might take the form of an algorithm and be put into the form of a flow chart, and might look something like the one on the following page. With this kind of thinking going into a presentation, your goals will become clear to you and your opponent, and you will do a better job of presenting what you are trying to accomplish. You can have prepared the most logical, factual and reasoned information to prove the worth of your goals, but, unless you communicate it to your opponent in a way that is both understandable and adequate, it will be of negligible value to you as a negotiating tool.

The Importance of Language

One of the more disheartening effects of misdirected results in negotiation is the failure to understand one's failure to communicate correctly. Another stems from an inability to control an overwagging tongue. Both of these failures are perhaps best illustrated with some quotes from Lewis Carroll's "Alice":

> "Then you should say what you mean," the March Hare went on.
> "I do," Alice hastily replied, "at least—at least I mean what I say—that's the same thing, you know."

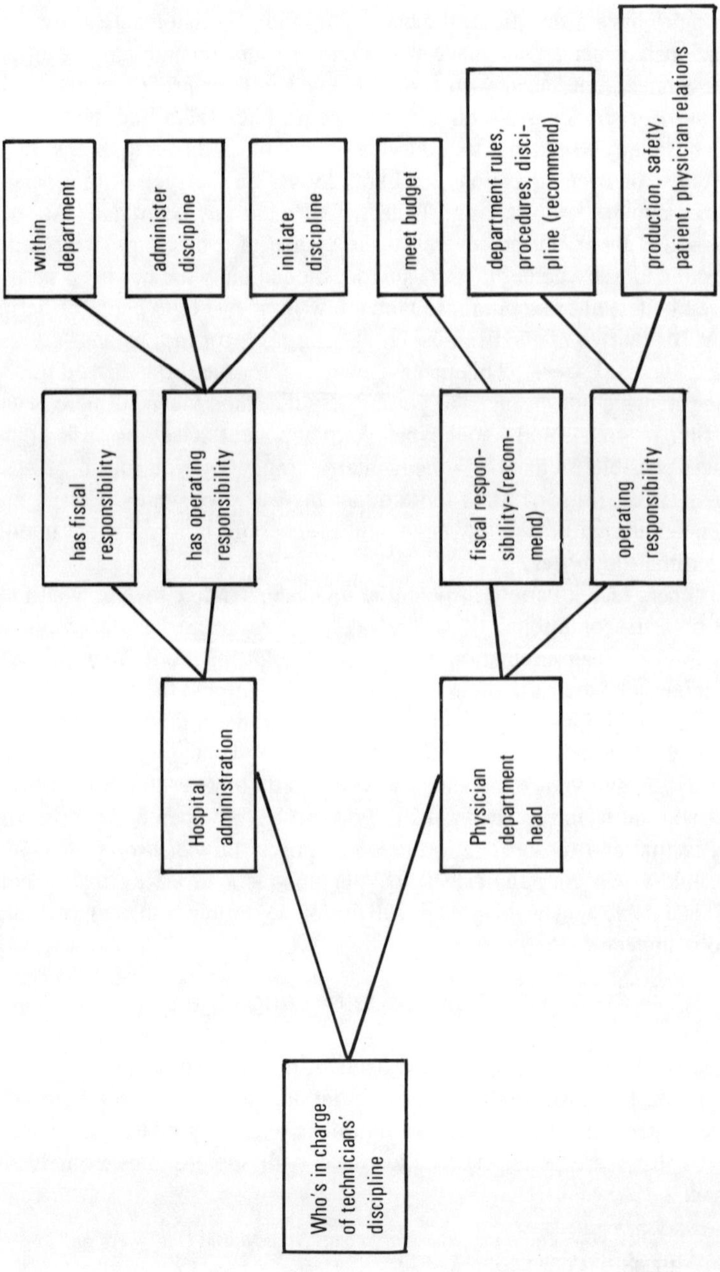

Who's in charge of technicians' discipline
Hospital administration
Physician department head
has fiscal responsibility
has operating responsibility
fiscal responsibility-(recommend)
operating responsibility
within department
administer discipline
initiate discipline
meet budget
department rules, procedures, discipline (recommend)
production, safety, patient, physician relations

> "Not the same thing a bit!" said the Hatter. "Why, you might as well say that 'I see what I eat' is the same as 'I eat what I see'!"
> and—
> "When I use a word," Humpty Dumpty said, in a rather scornful tone, "*it means just what I choose it to mean*—neither more nor less."
> "The question is," said Alice, "whether you can make words mean so many different things."
> "The question is," said Humpty Dumpty, "which is to be master—that's all."

A good rule of thumb when negotiating is to use basic language, particularly when involved in difficult and complicated problems. One reason why: lexicographers tell us that over fourteen thousand different meanings can be implied or inferred if you limit your conversation to the five hundred most commonly used words in English. Present a position absolutely and simply and you are more likely to be successful.

Linked with the necessity for clear and meaningful language in one's negotiating conversation is perhaps the most difficult bit of self-discipline—listening. We should be able to hear ourselves as others hear us. What deep-seated attitudes does the listener perceive, not just from our words, but from the way we say them? Voice quality, thinly-disguised antagonism, translocation of terminology with which one is professionally comfortable to completely different non-professional areas, "hmmm's" "you know's" and "I mean's" and the like that indicate confusion or equivocation, impress a listener as much as do the actual words used. If you have several ideas to present at about the same time, first put forward the one of most interest to your opponent. As you present the pros and cons of the argument, the position that *you* want should be left to the last, both for impact and memory retention. Good use of clarifying adjectives will make the impression more lasting, and help distinguish your points from broad abstract statements.

With the use of ambiguous or ambivalent language, you place an opponent in the position of having to assume your meaning and intent. Too often, that assumption may not be correct. Then misunderstandings multiply. The best way to avoid an accumulation of misunderstandings is to spell out what you mean, even if it requires defining the words that you are using, as you use them. And, if you are on the receiving end of words that appear to be obvious, question their meaning—"Do you mean . . .?", or "If I read you correctly, you are saying . . ."—put your understanding of what seems to have several meanings into your own words and let your opponent agree or disagree. (At this point, if the clarification involves an important phase of the negotiations, put it in writing, and if your opponent agrees, have him initial it as correct. This will save time and insure against renegotiation if your opponent decides the issue was not settled to his advantage.)

Listening and Questioning

Work at developing the ability to listen and question. One can always do better when negotiating by paying attention to question marks rather than to exclamation points. Perhaps no skill is as necessary to successful negotiation as empathetic listening to the response from your question. It tends to compensate for other shortcomings in several ways.

- It gives your opponent an opportunity to ventilate feelings and to clarify the background for arguments, especially if your questions probe in the right direction;
- It helps you—at least it should—better understand your opponent's perspectives and strengthen your objectivity, which is most important in reducing the emotions that too often interfere with the clear thinking that negotiation requires;
- It gives you the time and opportunity to make sound judgements and develop workable alternative proposals;
- It demonstrates your sincerity and interest in what your opponent is saying about his position, and, incidentally, serves to enhance appreciation for your credibility and increase trust in you;
- It stops you from talking too much, especially at the wrong time. This can prevent you from making premature judgments, that are usually mistakes that can only jeopardize the outcome of your negotiations;

This emphasis on listening, as opposed to the usual process of hearing without paying attention, is the basis for the following series of commandments:

(1) Listen to *how* something is being said as well to its content;

(2) Avoid making any estimates (prejudging or anticipating) of what your opponent will say (too often we hear only what we want to hear);

(3) Let him finish whatever it is that he is saying, and above all, don't interrupt to challenge him with a confrontation;

(4) Don't allow prejudices or emotion to make you react—be aware of them, and master them;

(5) Don't approach a negotiating session intent on "getting down to business" right away. If your opponents begin with small talk or a tirade about something that may or may not have occurred, let them go on for a while. Whether its purpose is to relax or to vent, it can become the basis for more significant conversation;

(6) Listen for intonation and watch your opponent's facial and body expressions as reinforcement to what is being said. Understand and use body language. But be careful decoding it. Your opponent may reverse general principles to mislead you.

(7) At the proper time, ask questions to guarantee freedom from any doubts or obfuscation that appears. Either ask direct questions or rephrase statements to draw your opponent out;

(8) While observing your opponent's voice and body language, be conscious of your own. You are trying to project interest and sincerity.

(9) Listen carefully for "hidden meanings". Seek what is really most important to the person speaking. What is said isn't always what is meant;

(10) Above all, listen for content;

(11) Don't be afraid to take notes. You don't need a stenographic record, but you do need enough to jog your memory. Time tends to erase or change our perception of a conversation, and notes can reinforce arguments if questions come up about what was meant or intended;

(12) Because you are able to think more quickly than a person can talk, use this time to take notes and analyze what is being said as it relates to the problem under discussion.

The "art" of negotiating revolves around your speaking and listening skills. The conversations that you engage in both at and away from the table serve a dual purpose. First, of course, they support and promote your goals. Second, because a win/win result is the best outcome for negotiations between parties that have to live together, conversation should not exacerbate the feelings of *either* opponent. Be careful, then, of the semantics you use to illustrate your points. It cannot be stressed too often that what you say and how it is received determines just how well your positions and your goals influence your opponent.

Talking to Your Objectives

One problem that seems to persist in negotiations, particularly with physicians who always appear to act as though they are late for their next appointment, is that they think more of what they want to say than of the responses to what is being said. Use conversation to cross-fertilize both sides' ideas. Parameters exist for the goals of the parties, but the end result should be satisfaction with the outcome for both sides. Because most physician negotiations are interim arrangements of ongoing relationships, you have to spend time and effort to discover what will satisfy your opponent beside the tangible results that the two of you are discussing. The material results—duties, financial arrangements, responsibilities, results, etc.—are the obvious ends of the negotiations, but many times subliminal needs also have to be gratified. You will often find that satisfying these unstated needs of an opponent will make a closer realization of your goals less difficult. Some of the unstated needs that negotiators have include:

- to keep his or her job;
- to be promoted;
- to feel important;
- to be trusted and liked (not unusual for administrators);
- to be the object of kindness and consideration;
- to avoid tension and conflict, as well as insecurity and surprises;
- to work less hard while eliminating future trouble and risk;
- to be respected for general competence and so have a feeling of self-worth;
- to get the negotiation concluded and get on with work that to him may seem more important.

Appreciating an opponent's subconscious needs and the emotions that create them requires you to have the honesty to understand your own underlying needs. Work to: get and hold your opponent's attention by piquing his interest in your proposal; allay and eliminate his skepticism while establishing your credibility to gain his trust (in an ongoing situation, much of this emphasis will have been either established or devastated by your daily relationship, so don't depend upon a few sessions of negotiations to change adversarial feelings—know where you both stand); increase your opponent's desire to pursue your proposals or alternatives and eventually work out a solution of value to both sides.

What is being sought is usually backup or clarification of assumptions made in your internal evaluation of the opponent's statements. Those assumptions must be tested and revised on the basis of what is learned as conversation proceeds. What is being negotiated is not always clear, so the areas of difference must gradually be reduced into issues that are essential (prime goals) and non-essentials (side issues). Remember: to achieve a win/win solution everything on the table is "negotiable", meaning that while every effort will be made to agree on primary goals, the result may have to be modified from the ideal.

A good negotiator only reveals as much information as is necessary at any one time. The responsibility for expanding, clarifying or disputing that information rests with the opponent. One is faced with imperfect information, which unfortunately becomes the basis for assumptions. Giving partial information should not be viewed as lying, which to a seasoned negotiator is both unnecessary and dangerous because of the effect of lying on credibility. Likewise, early full disclosure is a poor and dangerous tactic because with all your ammunition spent, you've nothing left for negotiating material. You will have eliminated most of your potential areas in which to maneuver. That brings us back to validating assumptions made because of what our opponent has been saying.

Ask questions, of course, but not just off the cuff. Frame them in several ways so you get the clarification you seek. You can buy time to think through your questions: (a) easiest, and at the same time productive in clarifying what your opponent has been saying, is to ask him to "go through it once more, please"; (b) caucus, to discuss what may need clarification. If alone, find an excuse to leave the room or request time to think about the issues; (c) hold your tongue.—By remaining quiet after an opponent has just finished making what he felt was an excellent statement, you create the impression that he has said something that was apparently either unacceptable or too one-sided, which subtly puts the pressure on him to say something that will get a response from you. (d) rephrase your opponent's remarks, even to the point of including some contradictions, . . ."Did I understand you to say . . ?" or " . . If I heard you correctly, you are proposing . .". Once you have asked the question, stop and listen to the response before you ask another question. And, incidentally, work to make your questions require only one response at a time. Complicated questions elicit ambiguous answers. Questions, as well as one's narration, should be clear—extremely easy to understand.

The information presented in your conversation will be, in large part, the result of the data accumulated while preparing to negotiate. *Data* is made up of of raw numbers and facts, but *information* consists of meaningful coordination of numbers and facts. Information involves the addition of *values* to the data through thoughtful and perhaps innovative application of selection, interpretation, and rearrangement of the data. For instance, if you present the relationship of numbers of patients' visits to the numbers and types of procedures for specific days and time periods, and the costs or charges, you have accumulated data. But if you can, on a single page, present this data in statistical form that shows, for each of the past five years, percentages and relationships of patients, days of the week, costs and/or charges as they were related to the various procedures, with averages as conclusions at the bottom of the page, you have relayed information. You now have the knowledge and written material to make a logical proposal.

Two other distinctions here relate to *primary* and *secondary* information, and to *internal* and *external* information. Being aware of the distinctions, particularly when the information is being fed to you by an opponent, puts you in a better position to prevent misleading assumptions and misunderstandings. Any time you are on the receiving end of information that is being slickly presented, verbally or in data or graph format, question that information. As a matter of habit in negotiation, be prepared to question data. Don't accept it as fact or on faith, ask for the backup or primary data; the what, when, where, how, and who—and be prepared to recess and wait until you are given what you ask for. Then let your opponent wait until you have had the opportunity to examine it at your leisure. *Primary* information is originated and developed directly from sources in response to a specific need. *Secondary* information is exactly what the term implies—second hand. It is probably out-of-date, not totally or completely applicable to the present need or discussion, or collected at an earlier time by researchers with concerns quite different from those required by your current negotiation. Such information may also have been interpreted or otherwise tampered with by the original gatherers for their own purposes, or by subsequent users of the data before it was restructured to be presented to you. By the same reasoning, once you publicly present your primary findings, it becomes secondary information to anyone else using it.

The second information distinction concerns the differences between internal and external data sources. *Internal* information includes facts and other data collected within one's own organization—hospital, group, society, training institution, etc. This information is primarily, but not only, gathered to measure performance. *External* information, by contrast, is built from data collected outside one's immediate surroundings—what is happening within the healthcare provider framework and its subdivisions. This information can be more difficult to gather and to verify because of a variety of ego and professional jealousies, but it can well serve to establish bases for comparison "between them and us," and for guidelines.

Collecting and verifying information should not be done solely to reinforce preconceived ideas or prejudices. Asking the wrong questions, either of yourself or of your opponent, is probably the single most significant reason for misdirection or failure of valid information. Too often the question that is asked is either confusing or asked in the wrong way. We are constantly seeking the answers without paying enough attention to the questions. When framing your questions, ask yourself:

- *"Why do I require this information?"* It will help whoever supplies the answers to know *why* you need them. Understanding is vital to a successful search.
- *"How do I convert my information need into a question?* A precise statement of the need can usually produce precise answers for question development.
- *"How can I make my question more specific?* You may, at first, be asking too general a question.
- *"Will the answer that I receive be of value?"* Knowing the importance of the question and its priority to your goals can be a crucial assist to your researcher.
- *"Do I already have any information about the question I am asking?"* Knowledge of whatever background you already have will ease the problems of your researcher.

- *"How available is the information that I require?"* Common sense plus a knowledge of potential information sources can save time and misdirected effort.
- *"Can I answer the question myself?"* Again, the specificity of the question will avoid misinterpretation by your researcher.
- *"Is my real need for an answer or do I only need a source?"*

Phrasing your Questions

What your questions will, or should, be at any particular stage of a negotiation, is not something that can be predicted. Don't get the feeling that information will be unavailable before you even start. You should be ready to raise questions about anything, and be ready to fit the answers into your game plan for a negotiation or discard the line of questioning if it fails to advance your cause. The value of the information you collect lies in its application to your goals, not in the search. The time required to collect information, the cost of acquiring that information, and its ultimate value to the point(s) being made should determine your research.

Getting the best answers to questions correctly phrased is not enough—no answer is worth anything if it is improperly interpreted. Failures of interpretation can be reduced if you gauge the reliability of the source of the information, how the answers have been put together for presentation, and the ability of the individual receiving that information to avoid personal biases. How the information is presented can be crucial to its potential use.. Know, and appreciate how the information has been organized from data, facts, statistics, and hearsay. Consider it may well have been "*massaged*" by the information-grantor for his own purposes (government-prepared statistics, accountant-prepared data for either internal or tax use, and lawyer-interpretations of codes either for internal or court use, are examples of preparing data for specific reasons—which is why I strongly suggest that you always ask to see the original data or backup information that supports the charts or graphs that have been put on the table). Correct and positive interpretation will depend upon your ability to perceive how the information has been massaged if indeed that is the case.

For example, if you request a budget increase for additional staff, the board of directors may be concerned with the quality of the services of the department before and since you took over. The following information is correct, but the massaging is evident.

Presented this way, if your estimates are correct and you have estab-

	1976	1977	1978	1979	1980	1981	(est) 1982	(est) 1983
Patient contacts	16,007	17,250	19,000	19,500	20,000	22,500	25,000	28,000
Procedures performed	24,000	26,000	26,535	26,700	26,765	29,000	30,000	32,500
Employees	27	27	28	28	28	28	28	30

% increase: 1976-83
Patient contacts — 74.92%
Procedures performed — 35.42%
Employees — 11.1%

lished your credibility with the members of the Finance Committee and the board, it is clear you will require additional staff to maintain the quality of service for which the department has been commended by the JCAH since you took over. Now, look at the same information graphed by the hospital administrator's finance officer, who wants to use the money you are asking for somewhere else in the hospital budget (graph A), and how you might present the same information in similar form (graph B): With the administration graph, the trends in patient contacts, procedures performed and employees on staff are relatively flat. This suggests that everything is moving along well with no real need for additional personnel. By contrast, your graph accentuates the increases in patient contacts and procedures performed while the personnel indicea remain almost static. The difference in the Finance Committee's perception is due to the scales that are used. When you are on the receiving end of this kind of presentation, pay close attention, view it with a more than healthy skepticism. With any statistical presentation, fall back on the well-known adage that "figures don't lie, but liars (figuratively, of course) figure." No matter how well someone uses and presents information, information is not the offspring of an exact science, and all the massaging of what may be accumulated pseudo-scientifically will not make it exact. But, you cannot ignore information put before you because it was subjected to the manipulations of a masseur. If it is ignored, it is of no value to you for refutation. To be of value, it must be taken into account and questioned.

Listening and questioning, strategies and tactics aside, will bridge the

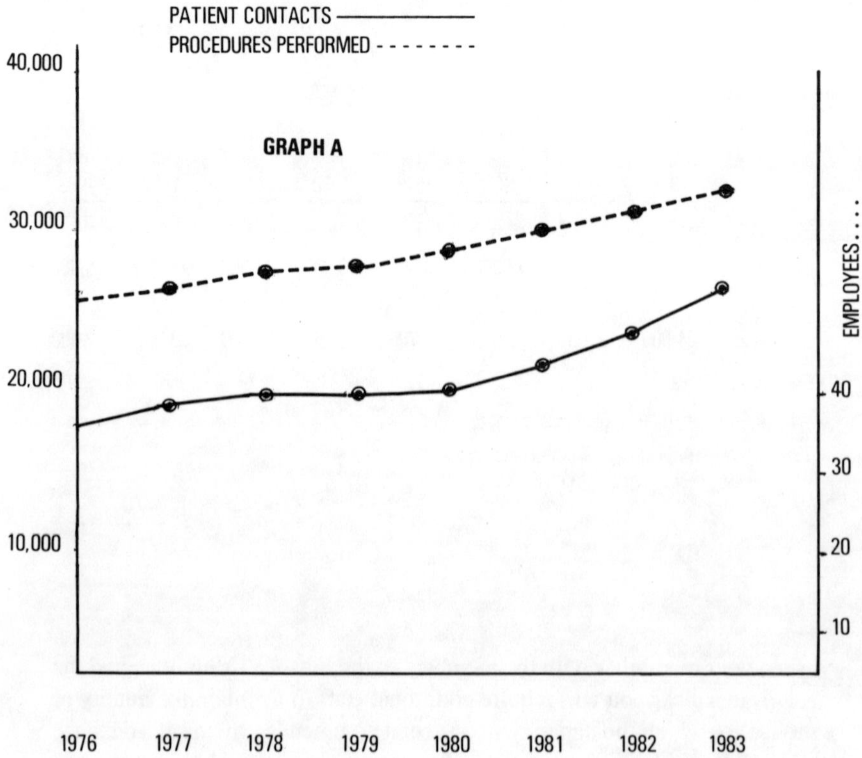
PATIENT CONTACTS
PROCEDURES PERFORMED
GRAPH A
40,000
30,000
20,000
10,000
EMPLOYEES....
40
30
20
10
1976
1977
1978
1979
1980
1981
1982
1983

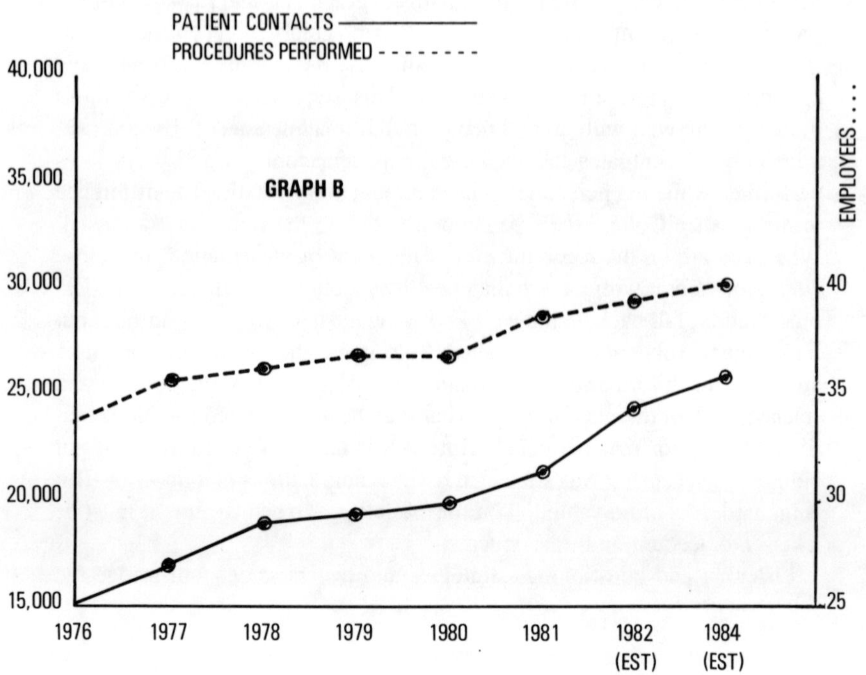
PATIENT CONTACTS
PROCEDURES PERFORMED
GRAPH B
40,000
35,000
30,000
25,000
20,000
15,000
EMPLOYEES....
40
35
30
25
1976
1977
1978
1979
1980
1981
1982 (EST)
1984 (EST)

chasms of potential misunderstandings and on the road to win/win results. With a better understanding, you can develop support for elements of an opponent's arguments to which you have minor or no objection, which sets him up for a *quid pro quo* that will be of benefit to your goals. Care must be taken in both asking and answering questions. Questions are difficult because they usually have to be answered at the time they are asked. You must answer, unless you can fall back on the complexity of the question so that you have to bring additional data to another meeting. Or, as a negotiator, you can escape answering quickly by saying you have to have time to study this data or to get approval from your principals. These methods may allow you to gain time to collect information or rebuttal ("it is beyond my authority"). But if you need some time to either fully understand the question or just think how you want to answer, it is permissible to give yourself a few seconds to think about your answer. Recognize, too, that some questions do not deserve answers. Ignore them and go on with whatever you were saying, or change the subject to something else that has meaning for your goals. Recognize, also, that sometimes touchy or bad parts of questions are better left unanswered at that moment. In such cases, answer the part that doesn't give you any problems with as extended and rambling an answer as you can, in hopes that the rest of the question will be forgotten. Or, as previously suggested, ask why the question was asked ("I don't understand what you are asking") or ask for an explanation of the words that you are not sure of. (One *caveat* for you to keep in mind: if any questions or issues are postponed, be sure that you keep a record of those that are pertinent to your goals so that you can raise them later in the negotiations. *Don't* leave those discussions to the very end or they will either receive short shrift or be passed over to your disadvantage.

One of the pitfalls that negotiators, and particularly professionals who are not adept at the process, have to avoid is being afraid to admit that they may be wrong or not completely versed in the subject matter being discussed. This kind of false pride can only lead to manipulation by an opponent. Don't feel threatened just because you ask for clarification. You are at that table negotiating either for yourself or for others, and to allow an irrational bogey of imagined embarassment to interfere with going after your fair share or your just returns is an obstacle that you can do without.

Preconceived impressions and emotional attachments must constantly be examined in the light of current available evidence. Such awareness has to be maintained because it is, unfortunately, in the nature of human relationships, particularly when analysis of one's perceptions of personal attitudes are involved, to follow Newton's Law of Inertia: *if something is allowed to remain undisturbed, it will continue on as before unless it is acted upon by an opposite force*. "Don't confuse me with facts," cynically protects the mind from positive solutions through negotiation. A skeptical but sincere examination of the potential pluses and minuses of situations should be part of the negotiator's tools.

The Total Message

When questioning and listening, gestures and inflections help get one's message across. Failure to merge all these efforts to communicate can result in a breakdown of information. Gestures, subject to earlier *caveats,* may be interpreted as either defensive or offensive by an opponent who takes them at face value. Some examples of gesture interpretation: avoiding eye contact may imply stress, anxiety or fear; chain-smoking may indicate anxiety; surreptitious mouth-covering may denote lying or avoidance; palm-steepling may show smugness, "my mind's made up and you can't change it;" increased eye-blinking and/or head tilting and leaning forward may show that your opponent is trying to follow what you are saying closely. Other signals, including the arms-over-chest, crossed legs, and leaning back with one's chair may or may not be significant. Be careful in putting too much faith in the interpretation of gestures—your opponent may be playing games.

Listen carefully to your opponent's voice. Under stress it may waver or increase in pitch. Be aware of words that may misinform such as: "Yes, but . . .," "Honestly, I . .," "By the way . .," "Truthfully, I . .," "Before I forget . . ." These statements should be signals for you to listen for either what your opponent is trying to conceal or minimize—he is being less than honest. Receptivity to both verbal and non-verbal communication doesn't come from reading books. Practice is the best way to increase one's sensitivity to negotiating skills.

Outright disagreement with an opponent's statement, harsh criticism, and gleeful indication of a mistake will usually only alienate him. Such actions take on the appearance of a personal attack and demand some kind of face-saving to assuage his ego. It would be better to create an excuse as an "out" to correct what may have been an incorrect view or conclusion: "I would have felt the same way you do if I hadn't read Dr. _____ 's article in the *New England Journal* a few weeks ago; or "Could one of your staff have misinterpreted the _____ figures in preparing them for you? My information, covered here in _____ is that _____." A series of well-planned questions can point out the loose thinking in an opponent's stand. These will usually be "Why?" questions. Or, you may ask questions that force a choice by asking "either . . . or" answers. Finally, if you can ask questions that create a "yes" atmosphere, the agreement you seek may come more easily.

Summing up the inherent problems of communication in the negotiation process, remember to:

- **Work at listening.** Profitable listening is hard work. You must be listening for both the *how, what* and *why* of your opponent's content. Purposeful attention means that through eye contact, posture and expression you are telling the speaker that you are with him and that what he is saying is being treated with the importance it deserves.
- **Keep your mind on what is being said**—don't let your thoughts rush ahead to counter arguments. There will be time enough for rebuttal or agreement.
- **Use your ability to think faster than you can listen by trying to anticipate**—without making assumptions—by asking "What is he getting at?" or "What's his point?" Be able to summarize what is being said so that you will be able to play it back to him.
- **Don't let antipathy become a block to your listening.** Premature judgments will create trouble for you somewhere down the line.

People have a tendency to listen only for facts. By listening with empathy you can also sense a speaker's *feelings.* The tone of voice, the postures and gestures, the timing of interpretations into the subject matter, the way proofs are offered can all be clues to how he feels about a subject. If, for example, he is overproving his point, it indicates that he already anticipates resistance from you or that he may be uncertain. If you are impressed that your opponent's feelings are an important facet of his presentation, occasionally interject: "Do I understand you to say that . . ." or "I gather that you approve (or disapprove) of . . ." filling in the attitude you believe he is expressing.

- **Watch out for controversial issues.** We often react to such issues without putting them through our intellectual wringers and fail to fit them into the context of what is being said. Wait until the meeting is over before you exercise your idealogical prejudices pro or con.

- **Listen, then wait a few moments before taking up the conversation.** It is too easy to become so interested in what is being said the need to immediately react and continue the dialogue takes over. The more emphatic your views or reactions are to a subject, the more likely you are to perpetrate this negotiating error. Don't tune out the content of what is being said in order to plan what are usually adversary retorts to only a portion of what was said. Instead, postpone the temptation to make assumptive conclusions until your opponent has had the opportunity to complete a statement. If you come right back to disagree, not only will you possibly antagonize him, you will undoubtedly find that you hadn't heard all of his position because you were so busy thinking of your comeback.

- **Think through the questions you put to an opponent.** Bear in mind the legal profession's truism that you should only ask questions (if possible) for which you know the answers. Questions have to be fully understood by both questioner and responder to be effective. Again, do not be afraid to ask "What do you mean by . . ." or to explain what you mean when words can have different meanings. Understand, too, that some questions do not require answers. Such questions may be ignored or require only an "Uh-huh", "Well . . ." or "No." A circuitous partial answer may deflect the original question. You can also ignore the question and ask another one. To gain time you can always ask him to restate the question, if it is especially difficult, or not to your advantage to answer in the way it was originally put. Should your opponent continue to push for an answer, and you are finally up against the wall to reply, answer, but with some qualification. "Well, depending upon . . ." or "My feeling is . . ." If you qualify your answer, no one can later accuse you of an untruth if later you adjust your position.

- **Play dumb as an effective last-ditch defense against an opponent who may be more experienced or better prepared than you.** There are not many things that take place at a negotiating table that can be more frustrating than trying to resolve issues with someone who either cannot, or will not, understand. Rephrasing out of context, requesting repetition with an "I don't understand . . ." or just sitting and looking at an opponent after he has made his point can be helpful—if not used too often.

8
VALUE SYSTEMS ANALYSIS

Man's judgements of value follow directly his wishes for happiness—they are an attempt to support his illusions with arguments.

Sigmund Freud

Negotiators should understand the broad value systems that shade their actions.[1] Each individual works his way through life with different expectations and different needs. And, as expectations and needs change, so do the individual's values.

As the principal or spokesperson for a set of objectives at a negotiation, you must understand your own values and attitudes. It also is necessary to determine as well as you can your opponent's values. Obviously, you must make some assumptions about your opponent at the outset. Those assumptions can be verified, or changed, as the negotiations proceed, as you observe him in action. As we noted earlier, the way to determine "where he is coming from" is to listen to his choice of words and watch his body language. Be sure to ask for the "why's" behind his statements. They will help you determine value levels. As you will see from what follows, once you have some idea of your opponent's value levels, you will be more effective.

---

[1]The material in this chapter is based upon lectures delivered at AMA Department of Negotiations seminars by Charles Hughes, Ph.D. and Vincent Flowers, Ph.D., principals of the Center for Values Research, Inc. 13771 North Central Expressway, Dallas, TX.

Most people operate at both primary and secondary value levels. If you observe more than one value level in your opponent's attitude, try to determine which seems to be most natural to him. If he exhibits several value levels as he goes along, they will most often be either values in the system that correspond to the even-numbered or odd-numbered levels we are about to explain. Seldom will a person simultaneously combine an even- *and* odd-numbered level. In any case, the concept developed by Drs. Charles L. Hughes and Vincent Flowers can be an effective tool toward appreciating how to meet and understand an opponent. Use it only as a tool—don't expect it to be a panacea. The basic assumption of the Value Systems concept is that people's values are not "right" or "wrong," but that they are individually "different." Each person reacts to a value level that is right for him at that period of his existence.

Value Systems Analysis developed practical applications, and assigned word labels which are based upon the theories of Dr. Clare Graves.[2] Before describing the value systems levels of human existence, let's consider the theory behind them.[3]

> "Unlike most "Values" frameworks, Graves' theory postulates physiological correlates of the psychological changes in people and speculates that people progress through consecutive levels of "psychological existence" from birth, according to their opportunities for acquiring and assimilating knowledge and exercising and developing their talents.
>
> The theory states that the psychology of mature human beings is an unfolding process marked by the progressive subordination of older lower-level systems to newer higher-level value systems.
>
> Mature persons tend normally to change their psychology as the conditions of their existence change. Each successive value system is a state of equilibrium through which people pass on the way to other states of equilibrium. In a particular value system, individuals have a psychology which is particular and peculiar to that value system. Acts, feelings, motivations, ethics, preferences, and thoughts which come about are behaviors one must adopt in order to solve his problems at that level of existence.
>
> However, people do not automatically move up to another level of existence, They may not be genetically or constitutionally

[2]Clare W. Graves, "Levels of Existence: An open system of Values," *Journal of Humanistic Psychology,* Fall, 1970.

[3]Charles L. Hughes and Vincent Flowers, "Value System Analysis (TM) Theory and Management Application," Center for Values Research, Inc., Dallas, TX., 1978.

> equipped to change in the normal upward direction when the conditions of their existence change. They may move, given certain conditions, through a hierarchially ordered series of behavior or value systems to some end, or they may stabilize in any one or combination of value systems in the hierarchy.
> Individuals may show the behavior of a value system in an active or passive manner, or they may, under certain circumstances, regress to a behavior or value system lower in the hierarchy. Thus, people live in a potentially open system of needs, preferences, and aspirations. In any one value system they have only the behaviorial degrees of freedom afforded at that level. Therefore as their societies develop, members of the societies must subordinate old values and behaviors if ever they are to develop new values and behaviors appropriate to new levels of existence.

Following a brief description of the value system will be equally brief suggestions for the most effective way to deal with opponents who appear to personify that level in their meetings with you.

Value System 1—Reactive

Infants and some people with advanced brain deteriotation or brain damage are assumed to have no system of values. Such persons react to conditions of hunger, pain, discomfort, warmth and apparent or real sympathy, but they do not respond to individuals as personalities. For our discussion, it is sufficient to realize the condition exists.

Value System 2—Tribalistic

People in this value system have deep need for stability, protection, and tradition. Loyalty to a leader, and familiarity and adherence to the customs of the group are their primary characteristics. Tribalistic individuals are essentially interested in feelings of security and continuity, satisfying and serving their existence by adopting the standards set by the authority figure they recognize. Tribalistic people do not make decisions as negotiators and their abilities to think imaginatively are limited; any variation from the instructions given them by their leader will require adjournment so they can report back and get further instructions.

Should you be put into a situation of negotiating with a level 2 individual, be self-assured and decisive and take charge. While you may express your concern for the group that the 2 is representing, you must speak with authority. You cannot, in any way, denigrate that opponent's leader. Logic and substantive arguments will not make the 2 switch loyalties. The most you may accomplish will be to have him recognize you as a negotiating chief while remaining loyal to his own leader. Project an image of a group leader who is not necessarily in conflict with his own leader, and make sure, through repetition and having him repeat to you, that he accurately and unmistakenly is able to pass on your position to his leader who makes the decisions. Meet 2's face-to-face, and preferably in meetings on their home ground so they will be as comfortable as possible in a difficult situation. Gain their trust.

Value System 3—Egocentric

People in level 3 will come across as aggressive and argumentative. They are individuals who have become aware that they can move away from the group and the leader-worship, and that this new freedom symbolizes their need for survival in an antagonistic world. Such people are extremely concerned with maintaining "face." They are more concerned with proving themselves than with the results of a negotiation. Extremely egocentric, they believe they have the right to do or be anything they wish in order to satisfy their pride, greed, envy, or need for survival. Power and ego satisfaction are their primary concerns. "The Hell with you" is their predominant attitude. They are restive, ruthless, testy and obstinate.

When negotiating with a 3, you will have to act more egocentric than he. He only respects power, and particularly the implication that physical power is there waiting to be used. However, because of the "saving face" syndrome of the egocentric, he should *never* be "put down" or criticized with anyone else present, unless you want an enemy for life. To be effective with a 3, eye-to-eye communication, preferably on a one-to-one basis, is essential. A 3 does not like to have things put in writing, would rather work from a verbal, person-to-person arrangement. A 3 must be convinced that, as a negotiator, you are either as powerful or more powerful than he, or he will try to trample all over you. Solutions to problems must, of course, be satisfactory to your goals, but must be stated so that he feels that he has made some points as well. With a 3, respect is earned only through the exercise of power.

Value System 4—Conformist

Perhaps the best label for a level 4 individual is "bureaucrat." A 4 believes he must discipline himself according to the rules of his universe.

only allowing himself to live by the blacks and whites set by those rules. Conformists are upset by ambiguity, preferring a straightforward no-nonsense negotiation. The 4's individual ego will not become a factor in his across-the-table behavior as long as the negotiation follows a formal pattern, and he does not have to deviate from his instructions. He will act inflexibly because he has been locked in by his supervisor's directions and interpretation of the rules of that group. "Should" and "ought" are keys to a 4's thinking. "Why not . .?" will only result in a parroting of the rules as the 4 understands them.

Negotiating with a 4 requires that you avoid being casual or overly friendly. Be clear about what you expect from him and his organization in the negotiating format, and negotiate in a consistent, organized, structured, and businesslike manner. Stick to an agenda and be prepared to overwhelm the 4 with facts, reports, statistics, laws, and regulations—preferably in writing. "Good faith", demonstrated by your sincerity, your honesty, and your credibility, will help to open up a 4 and allow you to present the correctness of your position in an organized manner. Put as much as you can in writing—memos, understandings, intents, minutes, etc.—being sure that your 4 opponent gets copies.

When negotiating with a 4, be sure to present a logical and reasonable explanation of your position to assure him that everything being proposed corresponds to his "book" and published policies. Do not allow inconsistencies to sneak into your presentation, or leave out any details, or he will lose sight of your "mutual" goals. Do not expect that 4 to respond to originality or creativity. Conformists expect to work within an SOP (standard operating procedure). As a result of following orders, the 4 responds to both approbation and fear of possible disciplinary punishment. To deal with a 4, you have to know the book better than he does.

Value System 5—Manipulative

Coming from value level 4, where the individual is the creature of his environment, we come to level 5, where the individual makes every effort to control his environment. (How better to portray both hospital administrators and surgeons?) Materialism, competition, enterpreneurial drive and gamesmanship are the tools of these "wheeler dealers." Winning is the name of the game. You may remember a movie in which James Garner played a Texas con man on the loose in New York. Wheeling down the boulevard, he was asked why he had to keep accumulating money. His reply was classic 5, "The money is not important. It's just a way to keep score." The 5's do not follow a consistent pattern. They will use whatever argument gives them the strongest position at a particular point in time, shifting from logic to emotion to bluster, and seldom laying all their cards on the table. Given the proper bait, the 5 can be imaginative, innovative, and cooperative as long as he can get the credit and feel that he has manipulated you to your goals. They will work within the rules as long as they are clearly spelled out.

Staying even or perhaps getting ahead of a 5 will require a good deal of "stroking" to show the 5 what the payoff can be for him. It will require a lot of flexibility on your part. Constantly review your agenda to guarantee everything you're concerned with is discussed. Negotiate aggressively and enthusiastically, openly confident with what you are doing because the 5 will leap to take advantage of signs of weakness or indecision that might give him an advantage. Your problem with a 5 will be discovering his *real* position which may be considerably different from what he expresses as his objectives. Always keep some potential concessions in reserve, knowing that one facet of his manipulative makeup is to "one-up" you. And, *do* keep detailed notes of all your meetings and conversations, for later use and reference because your 5 is so busy maneuvering that he will have a tendency to forget or deprecate some agreements after second thoughts. Build your presentation around the ways that settlement will benefit him personally and his organization.

Value System 6—Sociocentric

Sociocentrics are the "do-gooders." Getting along with the members of their peer group is more important than being successful. Harmony, interpersonal relations, cooperation within the group, and concern for "people" are the signs by which one can recognize the sociocentric person. The 6's see power structures as unnecessary because they serve to put people down. The relationships between people, how people help each other cope, and the hypothesis that society and the amorphous ideal of humanity pervade the thinking of the sociocentric. At no time during meetings with a 6 should you mistake this concern for the masses as weakness. He could kill you to make you see the light.

Negotiating with a 6 requires appeals to emotions rather than the usual litany of facts, figures, and logical arguments. The 6 can become difficult to move from his idealistic perceptions, so your best approach is to appear to share his concerns for people. Once established as a kindred soul, your arguments should be built around the ways that your proposals will lead to improved realtionships. Work to help the 6's reach consensus within their group. As an assist, while talking to the group as a whole, emphasize your points to the different members of the group as individuals. Consider dressing the way the 6's do, and make the meeting place and atmosphere as casual as possible. Working with sociocentrics can be difficult if you have become accustomed to following your own or mutually arrived at agendas, because their attention and expressed interests have a tendency to wander. Patience, and your often expressed concern for the welfare of whatever group is at risk (remember "patient care"?), and the opportunities for improvement that your solutions will develop should become the central themes for your discussions. Tying 6's down with detailed memos, long written documents and legalisms can be difficult. They operate on emotion and trust, but 6's have to be made to go beyond a handshake. Although you may have verbally agreed on something that will benefit many, the 6's you are negotiating with may not be the people who will put it into practice—and others cannot always be depended upon to honor a verbal agreement.

Political manipulators try to lead you down a primrose path with their alleged concerns for the down-trodden. Dig for the hidden agenda, whether it be power, personal advancement or whatever, and stick to your agenda with as few major concessions as possible until you are able to pierce the facade that may be there. Drop hints about benefits that may accrue to them and watch and listen very carefully. Stay relaxed with the 6's and stroke them, even though it may be tiring.

Value System 7—Existential

Perhaps the most interesting and challenging opponent you will meet will be the individual who has moved through all the earlier levels to a present set of values. The existential is a true individual. He is not the tough, aggressive 3, nor the wheeler-dealer 5. Existentials are creative, adaptive and decision-oriented individuals who have developed a high tolerance for ambiguity and for people whose values and ideas differ from their own. In many particulars they have become the synthesis of levels 5 and 6. They are concerned simultaneously with getting ahead and with the betterment of their fellow man, while being able to see manipulation for its shallowness and conformity for its thought-restrictiveness. Sevens are people whose favorite question is "why?". Sevens see problem-solving as a challenge. Flexibility in working with people, and challenges that require imaginative and responsible solutions are the forces that drive the existential. Having been involved in all the developing levels, the 7 will not spend much time playing the psychological games of the lower-value opponents, although eminently qualified to meet them on their own levels. As an actual or potential 7 do not be fearful of being open and honest; work for solutions, letting your imagination—and your opponent's—flow free.

Work with a 7 as with an equal. "These are "our" problems," "this is how the problems have developed," as well as "here are several approaches to problem A," will develop a working relationship and capture interest. Any attempt at gamesplaying will disinterest the 7, and lose his interest in problem-solving to the point that he may leave the negotiations because they are not productive. Solutions are what the 7 is looking for, and no alternative which might lead to a mutually satisfying result should be overlooked. However, once agreement has been reached and finalized, do not expect the existential to spend much time implementing the agreement. He is already looking for new problems to solve. Execution and administration, as far as the 7 is concerned, can be left to the 4's and 5s.

The successful negotiator understands that negotiations will not always be logical or follow a prescribed pattern. Working with Value Systems analysis can be a useful tool for a negotiator willing to take the time and effort to make its precepts advantageous. However, it is but one of the tools available to a negotiator. Understanding the principles that are expounded elsewhere in this book in combination with an understanding of other peoples' value systems, motivations and behavioral patterns can lead to better results than blundering and demanding "non-negotiable" proposals. Few people that you will meet across a negotiating table operate solely within a single value system. They are combinations of several systems. There will usually be a primary set of values with one or more backup levels. Value system classification indicates *why* people may act as they do, as opposed to the "what" or behavior pattern in which they operate.

For example, an individual who wears a suit and tie to work every day manifests a behavior pattern that reflects a value system. The question becomes "why" he wears that suit and tie. The 2 dresses this way because he was told to do so or because that is the tribal ritual of the group. The 3 may dress that way because it makes him feel "cool" and better than others. The 4 wears a suit and tie because people "should" and because when people work together they "ought to" look "right." The 5 hopes the suit and tie will impress others and make him look successful. The 6 does not want to look different or cause any hard feelings (Have you noticed that most non-conformist 6's tend to dress in the same uniform?) Finally, the 7 wears a suit and tie because it feels good and he wants to. If it didn't feel good or make sense, he would dress differently.

Because of the emotional cast that often pervades a negotiation, it is important that in countering or meeting opponents' value systems the negotiator recognize that he must act in a manner that will be effective with those opponents. Promises or exaggerations that are not intended to be fulfilled can make that opponent feel cheated or put upon, ruining the investment of extended time that negotiations require. When necessary, be as explicit as possible, and particularly when formulating the language of the final agreement, be sure that the words say what was intended. Protect yourself. Remember that everyone's value system is correct for him at that time if he feels safe and content with it, and that it is not up to you to change your opponent. Remain flexible, and you should do reasonably well.

9

DEALING WITH THE SNAGS

> *From a strategic point of view it is important that the administrator recognize and use conspicuous outcomes to his own advantage, if he can, or develop tactics that prevent the other party from focusing on conspicuous outcomes that are undesirable.*
>
> *Dean E. Grant,*
> How To Negotiate Physician Contracts

An answer that seems relatively transparent to one negotiator will often seem obscure to the opponent. Yet, the end result of extended and involved negotiations, when studied dispassionately, seems so obvious that both parties should have been able to agree much earlier. The psychologically desirous solution normally directs us to search for the simpler answers and to avoid complicating factors. If the issues on the table are not complex, giving in to this easy way out may be the best way to conduct the negotiation. However, settlements are seldom easily reached, particularly in medical socioeconomics. The physician negotiator, for example, negotiating with an administrator, must always be on guard against being guided into a "conspicuous outcome" of obvious solutions in order to finish quickly and get back to doctoring. In such cases the warning signal will probably be a deluge of statistics and corroborating data that make obvious solutions appear inevitable. This is the time to lay back and question, to appear unable to absorb all that information. It will also be a good time to try to move to another issue because you will need time to study what has been presented so overwhelmingly well.

If your preparation has been complete, you should be able to answer an administrator's apparent objectivity and the seemingly impressive righteousness of any cause with your own credible research. Question and challenge! Demand complete backup for all the material, study it, then adapt it to your goals.

When the tide of negotiations is moving your way, you will have a better chance to achieve your more important goals. When, where, and how well you make the process work for you will probably decide the outcome. Understanding when to shift from an unproductive discussion or subject is as important as abandoning the uncompromising pursuit of an objective.

Thinking vs. Reacting

How an opponent views you and your agenda, as capable or inept and outrageous, is primarily how you are perceived. You have to begin with the focus that people are where they are because they will seldom be where you want or expect them to be. You may not agree with their biases or opinions, but, to negotiate, you have to understand them. And, before you can change their views, you must understand them. Difficult as it may appear to you or to your opponent, there usually is at least a kernel of truth or propriety in any conviction. These kernels are rarely the whole truth. Your job as a negotiator with specific goals is to persuade opponents to step away from their convictions, at least part way, in order to understand your perspective. Being argumentative will only make an opponent more emotional and more stubbornly committed to his convictions. What you are searching for is shared ground so that both can begin to agree about issues over which you previously disagreed. Too often discussions fail to join the issues—the parties talk about different things and fail to get to the heart of their disagreements. By failing to create mutually understandable common ground, opponents have a tendency to allow their tempers to rule. Angry people fail to think—they simply react. And, when they react, they normally do so in the direction of their beliefs, their dogmas, and their prejudices and are likely to make mistakes. Only through patient and explanatory communication can one open an opponent's thought processes.

Personal achievement—winning—too often predominates over the goal of mutual understanding. The exercise of raw power, rather than efforts toward mutual achievement, only creates stress that negates the ability to negotiate. Changing an opponent's perception of an apparent controversy from a negative to a positive attitude with some honest appreciation of your point of view can reduce some of the stress of a controversy. Strive to show your opponents the wisdom of your solution to a problem. They might welcome the opportunity to change their opinion which helps clear the air around the bargaining table and leads to a win/win solution.

The Importance of Perspective

The introduction of new perceptions and understandings is somewhat like standing in the middle of a bridge and looking at both approaches. Perception may begin with an appreciation that one has been taking a strictly black or white position, much as the picture that follows. Who or what do you see? If I first suggest an old woman with an outsized nose and jutting chin, wearing a scarf, can you also see a fancy young matron of the "Gay Nineties" with long eye-lashes who is starting to turn her head? Or, if I suggest a young woman with a fancy hairdo first, can you also see an unattractive, poorly-dressed older woman? Which is the "real" subject? Your first perception may make it difficult to visualize the other. But, in fact, both are "real." A little concentration, a changed perspective, and you are open to another view.

It has been said that the only constant in life is change. A safe assumption for any physician to make is that change, choice, and confrontations are the reality of managing our lives for tomorrow. The problem before a negotiator becomes the effectiveness of choice processes. Effective choices produce constructive challenges—ineffective choices only produce confusion and failure. But, change and choice-making produce anxiety, avoidance, annoyance, and anticipation, all leading to tension.

The tensions resulting from the presentation of a need for change in negotiations have to be relieved or they will end up defeating you. Letting tension take over to the diminution of interest in your agenda, gives your opponent an undeserved power that will only be to your disadvantage. *Status quo* is seldom a good defense against the choice for change; the tough fact that must be faced is that you and your opponent—as suppliers or factors in health care—are there to offer services to the public.

No negotiator worth his salt should let himself become incapable of adapting when the need for change has been fully documented and rationally presented. Failure to adapt to what on the surface first appears radical can occur when one becomes too involved in the practice, and unaware of the turmoil in today's healthcare field. Don't put yourself in that category through obduracy.

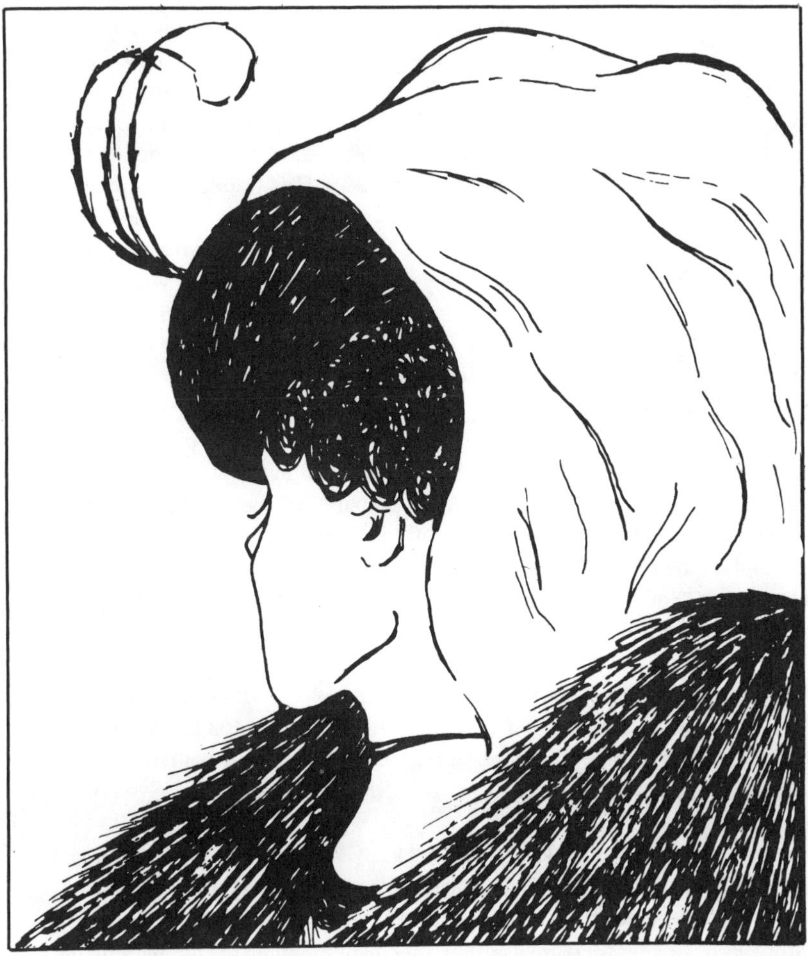

The Art of Compromise

If change is the core of the negotiation drama, then give-and-take will underline the importance of compromise, with reasonable satisfaction of the needs of the parties involved being the mutual aim. However, compromise should not mean that both parties concentrate so fully on satisfying the other's needs that they fail to properly present or advocate their own bottom line alternatives. A negotiator must always enter meetings with an opponent with an open mind. The agenda must be the guiding force in exchanges of information. Information exchanges, alternative approaches, potential solutions, must flow in both directions. The drama of negotiation must reduce the areas of disagreement between the parties. The worst thing a negotiator can do at any stage of the drama is to *demand* concessions from or to pressure an opponent in any fashion. Often a person who tries to pressure or demand unequivocally has a limited conception of the problem at hand and the potential solutions. To cope with an opponent who presents "non-negotiable" items, one either calmly offers a clear and reasonable suggestion to explore alternatives, or withdraws.

One can come to the negotiating table in response to an intolerable condition, or to correct or maintain a contractual agreement. Once faced with the certainty of negotiation, one's preparation and subsequent direction should be directed toward competition. Confrontation can only exacerbate and divide opponents. But competition in the stipulation of an ongoing relationship should not become an extreme effort to close the negotiation as *numero uno,* the winner. If that is the aim, we are back to looking at a confrontation of adversaries. Competition shifts to mutual concerns to evaluate and devise areas for mutual benefit—to a win/win conclusion. With both sides satisfied that each has done the best for the immediate future, the drama can end successfully. How well, or how poorly, you and your opponent achieve your goals will depend upon the attitudes you bring to, and maintain at, the table.

Attitude, consistency, flexibility, and knowledge will be your chief tools in the drama of negotiation. Consistency and flexibility need not be appositive ideas—one can be consistent in working toward one's objectives while being flexible in the ways they may be approached. The main theme of one's approach is to be positive, and to impress the opponent with your attitude.

Balancing what you want against what your opponent wants will make your negotiation manageable. However, reaching that point can be time consuming, and few physicians can afford to take too much time away from their patients, especially for what can be viewed as non-professional purposes. There will be those you will meet across the table who will be anxious to spend so much time reaching that clarification of issues—call it ventilation—through searching, denying, and explaining, that the resolution of issues becomes forced and less than satisfactory. (This is the bureaucratic approach.) Thus, one of the early subjects for discussion should be the time allotted for the total negotiation. Deadlines must be considered. For a contract re-negotiation the deadline is already in place. For negotiations of subjects with no specific end date, one should be set. However, as with most *dicta,* when talking about the negotiation process, times and dates are not immutable. A deadline should be considered only a tool for presupposing the end of a negotiation. If the conversations are moving promisingly, you don't sever a developing potential solution just because a predetermined point in time has been reached. Deadlines can be, and quite often are, put off and reset. But when patient care calls, when you believe that your opponent is waffling, and you want to finalize the negotiations, use the deadline. Ventilation cannot be permitted to go on interminably, because the longer that you permit an opponent to waste your time the less effective you become. Becoming positive about concluding a satisfactory agreement will increase the momentum toward conclusion.

When You Reach an Impasse

The decision to conclude can cause stalemate or impasse. Depending upon the stage of a negotiation drama that has been reached, during the ventilation sequence, or during hard (near final) bargaining, deadlocks can be either useful interludes or truly stressful situations. Make up your mind that you will use them when they occur. Do not let your feelings about an impasse take over and devastate your aspirations to the point where you: lose self-confidence; have guilt feelings that you either misinterpreted something said by your opponent or failed to satisfactorily clarify something; or think you might have to repeat the entire negotiation with a new opponent. Do make that deadlock work for you.

As an alternative to the settlement of issues, negotiators' persistence in refusing to move from what their opponents may view as unreasonable positions results in impasse. Deadlocks can raise the question of whether such a stand is the result of negotiating in good faith by standing on a principle, or whether the impasse is being used to stall or break off the negotiations. This is a time for patience and creativity. When you are up against a stalled issue, imaginative problem solving and flexibility can provide the impetus to movement.

When an impasse occurs early in the drama, it is usually easier to put the issue aside and move to another agenda item. Remember to keep some personal record of the tabled issue if it is important in your agenda, and be sure to bring it back to the table—before the time and pressure crunch to finalize the negotiations takes place. Another approach would be to continue negotiating, searching for alternative routes around the roadblock. These could include going back to the basics of the issue, talking to firm up the common grounds developed earlier. By emphasizing how little apart the two of you appear to be and the issues that have already been settled amicably (investment of time and effort) rather than the apparent differences leading to the stalled negotiations, interest in proceeding to search for alternatives may be developed. Repetition of the good things that have already taken place while downgrading the differences often loosens the strictures of an impasse.

Often a deadlock occurs because of a negotiator's hidden needs. Bringing out or discovering those unspoken but important personal needs and working out a way to satisfy or appease them, within reason of course, can create the momentum toward settlement. You may find that by going "off-the-record" either at the table or over a cup of coffee you can discover the reason for an adamant stand. Once in the open, the search for alternatives can proceed. An experienced negotiator will usually phrase his opposition to change or his position with care to leave opportunity for change. Here, careful listening pays off. That opponent may be taking that tough stand to impasse by overstating his convictions or positions to lower your expectations of favorable settlement. You can respond by changing the form of the issue that's deadlocked. Emphasize the favorable parts of his proposal and the discussion should begin again.

There can be times when all the goodwill, effort, and creativity you can muster fails to open the road to agreement. That may be the time to suggest bringing in a disinterested third party to mediate, fact-find, or arbitrate. When both parties agree to permit a third party to assist or decide their differences, they are obviously putting the burden of settlement on that party with the understanding that they will live with the outcome. A mediator will try to keep the parties talking, searching for a mutually acceptable middle ground. A fact-finder will listen to both sides, then make recommendations which the parties may or may not agree to follow, but may at least open new alternatives to discuss. An arbitrator will chair a hearing that allows each side to present its position and to cross-examine opponent's statements. Following this hearing, the arbitrator will issue a decision that is final and binding on the parties with regard to the subject being arbitrated. Mediators, fact-finders, and arbitrators, when used, should work within strict limits set out by the parties to prevent them from taking over all aspects of a negotiations or issues already agreed upon.

Should all efforts fail to break a deadlock, don't give up. Time has a way of leading to resolution of insoluble issues. As long as you have tried every option open to you, put it aside. Among the axioms that litter the writings of negotiators are two that every physician should take to heart: "Seldom will you get everything for which you go into negotiations," and "There's always tomorrow, when you can come back and try again if you still want to." One of the few results that cannot be accomplished through the negotiation process is turning a sow's ear into a silk purse.

Offers, Counteroffers, and Concessions

Too many people entering into negotiation assume that the only way to achieve a satisfactory solution is to open with an extreme, maximum position; in effect, a "take it or leave it" posture. They limit their options by presenting a smorgasbord "wish" statement of what they believe is best for them without considering their opponent's goals. By ignoring their opponents' positions, needs and intentions, they put themselves into the contrary conditions either of trying to force an unwilling acceptance of their ultimatum—with its attendant future of distrust and opposition—or permitting that opponent to decide which of those ultimatums they are willing to agree to while undoubtedly ignoring any discussion of what may be most important to the proposer. Too often, rejection is the result of such strategy.

Extreme openings normally receive extreme counter offers. Proposing extremes does establish the best wishes of a negotiator, while it conceals potential bottom-lines, and certainly can serve to inhibit a cooperative effort toward a mutually satisfactory solution.

Opening with a *fair* proposal shows intent to have a cooperative discussion. However, a more expectant but reasonable proposal may produce a more advantageous settlement. Remember—you and your opponent seldom will have the same definition of fairness. Also, making what one believes to be a fair proposal can induce a feeling in an opponent, particularly one who takes extreme positions, that he is being patronized. Offering a fair proposal, however, does emphasize a negotiator's interest in a win/win outcome. Obviously, the major problem that faces the negotiator who begins with a fair proposal is making it effective. For instance, if an opponent approaches you with a fair proposal, proceed with caution; it may be a concealed extreme. Begin by talking about it. If you are the proposer, talk about the intent and *mutual potential benefits* that can accrue to both sides before giving your fair proposal. This establishes some framework for your opponent's conception of how you view your proposal. Also, don't become self-righteous about the superiority of your notion of what actually is fair to both parties. Even though you have done your preparation well, and are convinced of the correctness and propriety of your proposal, let your opponent talk, while you listen. As the talks proceed, be consistent with your opening attitude of seeking a win/win agreement.

The drama proceeds after the parties have made their opening statements, established the opening reasons for their proposals, and have given further explanations in answer to early questions. The time has come to ask about the possibilities for modifying any of the proposals on the table. Depending upon how the mutual agenda was set up, you are at the point where, by careful listening and probing questioning, you should be getting some insight about his potential settlement limits, which of his proposals are most important to him (these may become the most difficult to concede), the correctness and amount of backup information available to him, and the kind of strategies and tactics he plans to employ. And you will be in approximately the same situation *vis-a-vis* your opponent.

This may be the time to corroborate your areas of potential agreement and disagreement. Based upon your preparation analysis, assumptions about your opponent's positions should be updated. This could be a good time to recess the negotiations in order to prepare yourself for alternative applications of arguments for your goals and reassessment of your opponent's proposals. Expected points of difference may have been clarified or exacerbated, with either position requiring a changed approach. Some of your opponent's information may include items that you did not consider in your preparation. Before you continue, you will want to study those differences. The information and conclusions that you reach as the result of this follow-up should fit in with whatever you have learned about potential settlement limits.

Working Toward Agreement

Back at the table, you are ready to enter the most time-consuming and complicated phase of the drama, working to agreement. When the aspirations of both parties are in limited disagreement, go to work for agreement. Resolve the differences that are apparent to both of you, get the settlement in a written memo, have it initialled by both of you, and put it aside. With the early areas of agreement out of the way, you are ready to work on your separate areas of concern and the mutual points of disagreement. Offers and counteroffers will, in effect, result from the search for concessions by both parties, as they work to develop alternative solutions to the subjects of disagreement. C. Northcote Parkinson, in his classic *Parkinson's Law* observed that ". . . the world is full of people who . . . knowing nothing of millions (of dollars) are well accustomed to think in terms of thousands (of dollars)." This can almost be accepted as a truism in the practice of negotiations. For some reason, when discussions get near or into the nitty-gritty many people begin to concentrate upon what appear to be insignificant details of a tentative settlement and neglect their larger goals. Use this to your advantage.

For example, the spokesperson for a medical group negotiating the purchase of property for their clinic and ambulatory surgical center was offering a sum much lower than was asked. Discussion revealed that the cost of title insurance and the inability to develop several plots of open land behind the property under consideration weighed heavily upon the seller's mind. One physician, after a quick call to his partners, offered to split the cost of the title insurance and other minor closing costs with the seller and to lease the undeveloped property, with an option to buy (at another low price), with the cost of surfacing the property for parking to be equally divided. Worries aside, the sale was consummated. Although the costs of the insurance and paving were minor in relation to the total cost and convenience of the original negotiation to the medical group, the additional offers were important to the seller. Without the alternative improvement of the lowball offer, the deal could have fallen through. By concentrating on what is important to accomplish your major goals, and listening carefully for the hidden agenda or peripheral emphases of your opponent, you may be able to end well above your bottom line.

Similarly, when negotiating with hospital administrations, peripheral issues or problems may be utilized as bargaining chips to get concessions that would otherwise be overlooked. For example, if there are nursing staff problems, an offer to help train nurses may create more cooperation in solving some of your problem areas with the administration.

Problem-solving becomes the name of the game at this stage of negotiations. However, one must be careful, particularly when negotiating in the healthcare field, not to confuse *conditions,* which are states of existence, with *problems,* which are situations that are solvable. Conditions sometimes might be unsatisfactory and require change but they are seldom conducive to quick resolution. Recognizing general conditions can lead to understanding and definition of the solvable problem situations. Understanding the conditions inherent in the management of a particular phase of health care requires an objective viewpoint and much patience. With patience and objectivity it becomes easier to define the problems that are caused by unsatisfactory conditions. An example: regulation is a condition which causes innumerable problems for health care personnel. How to charge imaginatively to receive reimbursement for outlays inadequately allowed for, how to provide services not in place when the regulations were conceived, how to utilize new procedures regarded as experimental and under-reimbursed to prove their value, how to maneuver between the conflicting regulations and interpretations of agencies concerned only with their limited authorizations and status in the competitive bureaucratic society, can open areas of mutual concern for discussion. Don't succumb to the frustration that "fighting city hall" creates.

Regulations, especially when issued by competing agencies administering the same or similar laws, are often contradictory. These contradictions are created by semi-independent bureaucracies often at the expense of those being regulated. "City hall" can occasionally be beaten, but it takes patience, persistence, and knowledge.

Perfect answers or solutions are seldom developed in negotiating sessions. Negotiators look for the best available solutions for the foreseeable future, knowing that as time passes any problems arising from a solution will be amenable to negotiation and solution. Problem solving requires that both parties mutually work to resolve the conflicts and differences that have surfaced during the negotiations. Mutual effort toward solution should be attempted before resorting to bargaining. Problem solving calls for a clear search for alternatives, free of any emotional overtones. "Have you considered . . . as an alternative to . . . ?" or "What do you think if . . . ?" can be leadins to opening a discussion of different approaches. Concentrate on looking directly at an opponent when proposing alternatives. An old First-Sergeant's trick that may be of use: when looking face-to-face, don't try to outstare eye-to-eye. Look at a point just above the other person's eyebrows. That way, your opponent feels that you are maintaining eye contact—but you avoid the pressure or stress of having those eyes boring into yours. Failure to maintain eye contact can give an opponent the impression that you either lack conviction or are insincere about your proposal.

Answering Your Opponent's Offer

You have three choices with offers, whether made directly or put forward as "consideration" suggestions. They can be accepted, turned down, or countered. Seldom should you immediately accept, unless it is truly "an offer that you can't refuse." Such proposals do not happen along very often, but if they do, take them. When an offer sounds too good to be true, the best tactic is to take one of two positions—consideration and study, or a "no, maybe." What you are doing is keeping your options open, while you look for potential shifts to advance more important goals, alternatives with a better gain, or compromises. To avoid having any doubts about whether you said yes too soon, putting an opponent's offer on the back burner with a need to study it or with a "no" is much better than grabbing something you are not sure of. A "yes" once given is difficult to take back. A "no," on the other hand, depending upon how it is presented, can be used to spur an opponent to rethink, rephrase, or continue to push for your acceptance.

Similar to a "no" could be a "yes, but . . ." answer. This serves to partially relax your opponent, giving you the opportunity to put forward alternatives more favorable to your goals. By appearing reasonable, you can make ambiguous and noncommital proposals that may defuse your opponent's proposal so that you can get on to items more in line with your objectives. Get back to the problem that started that particular discussion and reiterate the relevant facts, then propose several alternatives. Get your opponent to consider the quality as well as the quantity of the options you propose. Offering alternatives and discussing them with your opponent will usually result in something both can live with. If you are proposing an idea that is completely new to your opponent, don't push too hard at first. But, keep bringing it into the ongoing discussions. Like the old Chinese water torture of single drops of water continuing to fall on a victim, repetition softens the impact of a new thought. With that repetition, the "new" becomes a proposal your opponent has become used to. (However, should you become the object of this sort of tactic, your best protection is to find a way to put the proposal and drip tactic on the back burner. This can turn a "no" into a "yes, maybe . ." and give the proposer time to rethink both views on the subject. Stalling avoids outright rejection and provides time for restudy and reproposal.)

When faced with a turndown, ask: "What is unreasonable about these alternatives?" If your question is answered with the question "What is reasonable about your proposals?'', ignore it and use another question. ''I believe that I explained my suggestions fully. Is there any part you would want me to amplify, repeat, or explain?'' Should your opponent's objections appear sincere and reasonable, look to possible ways to adjust your alternatives, or present some other approach to your alternatives on the table. Should you persist in pursuing a single or the same alternative proposals you will only end in an impasse.

As we have seen, offers can be accepted, turned down, or countered. Any reasonable counteroffer can be perceived as a new offer. Counteroffers facilitate the negotiation process because the modifications create a willingness to continued discussion. What usually takes place is that either party finds a way to accept a part of the proposal, which has the effect of building an investment in both the continuing discussion and the final agreement. With offers and counteroffers comes the reality of concessions. My experiences with physicians have been that they too often regard the idea of compromise as unclean. Don't get emotional over the word! There is nothing indecent about compromise. Compromise, thoughtfully pursued, is not surrender, although you will find that hospital administrators are being taught that ''. . . compromising is not a substitute for effective negotiating skills and strategies.'' (*How to Negotiate Physician Contracts,* Dean Grant).

In the give-and-take of negotiation, concessions are part of the process. Look at it this way: If you are representing the hospital medical staff and one of your goals in negotiating with the administration is to have one-third of the members of the board of directors physicians, and one or two is all they are willing to concede, and that's the best you can do for now—grab it! When the other person appears to hold most of the cards—especially when you are after something he has always had, a compromise can achieve a reasonable amount of your objectives. If you can move the responsibility for decision-making to your opponent on the basis of your alternatives, you will come out ahead more often than not, especially if it is a matter of a simple division of available resources. (Put it to him to make the division, with you having first opportunity to choose which of the resulting parts to take.) You will find, over time, that most compromises are self-limiting. Either new problems, more pressing or disconcerting, come along, or time offers new opportunities for solution.

When getting into concessions the problem is one of when and how much. If you have built a few ''gimmees'' into your agenda that are of no importance to you, you will have something to give when the time for concessions comes. These expendables cost you nothing—and the same will go for your opponent—but will ease the way for both of you to get to serious give-and-take. However, don't just drop items without a *quid pro quo*. Failure to identify the need for mutually comparable "giveups" encourages an opponent to believe that you are weak and if he continues to hold out, he can impose his will without making any compromises. The most certain way to create compromise is to clarify the possibilities that exist through creative, alternative solutions. While designing concessions, one must constantly keep in mind the bottom-line objectives. Frame your concessions and those you seek from your opponent to fit your minimal limits. Perhaps the best way to handle compromises is to give way in small increments, while working to get your opponent to match your giveups in larger—or at least equal—increments while continuing to propose both good and not-so-good alternatives. Understanding what your opponent is seeking from the negotiation, what you want and must have, and what you are willing to concede can lead to agreement through problem-solving. Any other approach will most likely end up in stalemate.

Part of the problem is determining the trend of the compromises. Henry Kissinger, while still a Harvard professor, wrote that "If agreement is usually found between two starting points, there is no point in making moderate offers. Good bargaining technique would suggest a point of departure far more extreme than what one is willing to accept. The more outrageous the initial proposition, the better the prospect that what one 'really' wants will be considered a compromise."[1] While this approach may, in theory, work between two powerful opponents negotiating in the glare of media headline writers, it can create problems for parties dependent upon the outcome for their personal socioeconomic survival. Timing is the essence of concession-making. Cooperation balanced with a tough attitude can maximize the flexible approach that indicates a reasonably successful negotiator. A better strategy for most of the areas in which physicians will find themselves negotiating suggests an opening position greater than their expectations and bottom lines—but not as extreme as Kissinger suggests—that permits a lead-in to alternatives and offers room for maneuvering. In negotiating it is apochryphal that negotiators who make large initial and early concessions have a tendency *not* to do as well as their opponents because such actions give their opponents confidence and momentum, particularly if they are made without a *quid pro quo*. The best way to stay clear of making large initial concessions is to show your opponent that the positions you are taking are backed by solid factual or

[1]Henry A. Kissinger, *The Necessity for Choice*, 1961, Harper & Row, New York.

other support that is unquestionably valid. However, at times a large initial concession may be necessary. When that happens, you need not lose either momentum or the opponent's respect if you explain, fully and *ad nauseum* if necessary, your reasons for your actions. This will deflect any feelings of superiority on the part of your opponent because you are letting him know that you are not conceding because of either the weakness of your stand or a lack of self-confidence. Also, if you are put in the position of having to make that first large concession, do it on the basis that it will only take place if you also get something from him that may be important to your eventual success.

There will be times, when, to keep the movement toward agreement moving, trust and ingenuity must be put to work. Such times occur when issues present roadblocks because of the parties' insistence upon the "rightness" of their stands. Several alternative approaches may come in handy. One method is to divide the totality of the issue into its component parts and work for separate agreements on each of the parts, while keeping the original issue in mind. Separating an issue into resolvable components can be a challenge. If the parts become as non-negotiable as the main issue, nothing will have been accomplished. If, on the other hand, the breakdown into minor parts is effective, the parties can proceed with an exchange of ideas and concessions that will remove the main issue roadblock. Another approach to the big issue roadblock, particularly when the issue appears unresolvable, is to propose an intentionally ambiguous solution. While precise language is a goal to be sought in agreements in order to avoid problems during the term of an agreement, "constructive ambiguity"—as Kissinger calls it—can be useful in maintaining the continuity of a relationship. And, if such vague language does become a later problem, enough may have been learned by the parties in the interim that a means for settlement has surfaced.

Because the whole process of negotiation is verbal, the risk of misunderstanding what has been offered, counteroffered, or agreed upon is monumental, as previously discussed. To avoid the debilitating effect of either misunderstandings by you or your opponent on a final agreement, it is a good idea to present an offer or counteroffer in writing. Thus, there is less chance that the specific terms or conditions that are being proposed will be misunderstood, or, as too often happens when negotiations are sporadic or extended, forgotten. If it is inconvenient or impossible to present a written proposal with sufficient preparation, document it as a memorandum or in your notes. Be tactful. You don't want your opponent to feel that your trust in his ability to remember is diminished; you may even want to give him an edited copy of your notes. A written memo helps, especially when concessions are exchanged and agreements made. Taking the initiative and extra effort required to put things in writing pays off when writing the final agreement and settling differences that may come up in administering the signed agreement. Finally, the mounting accumulation of paper that documents the incremental agreements will help develop—in both you and your opponent—a feeling of investment and thus a potential sense of loss if negotiations break off. And it may allow a little nibbling for an extra tidbit. How well you can exact that last bit will depend upon how strongly your opponent wants a settlement and how your last offer falls within his range for a satisfactory settlement. If your opponent's need for agreement is not pressing, some small sweeteners, or hints of potential disasters, may serve to bring him around. The sweeteners will usually be giveaway items—ego-builders that make him look better to his superiors. The disasters would be negative consequences that your opponent would not want to see. Be aware—the same tactics can be used on you. Momentum and investment, when the crunch to close comes, judiciously applied, will move both parties' toward agreement. Although this is when there is more solid agreement than disagreement at the table, and a sincere interest in concluding the negotiations, it also can be a time when someone at the table tries to slip in some pet point that was bypassed earlier, or tries to renege on a point earlier agreed-to. This would be the last chance for a considerable period to alter the terms of an agreement that may exist, and the chance may be taken. However, this also can be the time for a firm "no" to see just how concerned the proposer is with his investment in the final outcome. Again, patience and firmness in negotiating should prevail.

10
CLOSING THE DEAL: THE LAST ACT

When you get right down to the root of the meaning of the word "success," you find that it simply means to follow through.

F. W. Nichol

The customer who is always right probably waits on himself.

Laurence J. Peter, Ph.D.

Finalizing a negotiation is your ultimate goal. Getting signatures on an agreement brings the curtain down on the drama. This is when your sense of timing tells you that neither you nor your opponent will be making any more concessions. All the alternatives have been explored, and you are both reasonably satisfied with the deals that have been made. Continuing to amplify points or tossing additional alternatives on the table can result in efforts to get back concessions.

When you feel that the time has come to close, you should summarize all the points agreed to—for which you both have initialled memos before you—making sure that, as you enunciate a point, you look directly at your opponent, then wait a moment. The pause will give him a last chance to disagree and evaluate any misunderstandings. This is the time when you can utilize the technique of presenting items as assumptions of agreement: "I'd suggest that we handle the details of payment by . . ." or "Your office will put the monthly data together so that . . ."

This is also the time to ask yourself whether the "final" offer really is the best you can get from—or offer to—an opponent. It is good negotiating strategy to always have some small give in reserve, a sweetener, if you will. But you don't have to give without pressure. When you are at the end of the road, say so. "This is my final, *final* offer to settle. I can go no further." Doing so tells your opponent you have extended yourself to your limit to meet them better than half-way, and puts an extra psychological value to your position.

As a physician, you are accustomed to getting effective results from your diagnoses and procedures. Don't fall into the mental trap of expecting a negotiation to solve permanently all the problems that caused the negotiations. Because people are party to the agreement you are concluding, there will be some areas of future disagreement. Where human and particularly contractual relations are involved, change is to be expected. Options should be built into agreements to provide for alleviation of disputes and disagreements so that the relationship can continue to work even under stress. Some form of due process or alternative action must be made available to the parties. For new and untried proposals, an escape clause can be agreement to try it for a limited period—six months, a year—so that if a better way surfaces, or it doesn't work out as planned, you go either back to the old way or renegotiate.

Agreements, particularly those made between hospitals and hospital-based physicians, may be subjected to third-party influence. If legislators or regulators are in the process of preparing restrictions during the period of negotiations, postponing agreement to further negotiation may be advisable. Without positive knowledge of the third party action, commitment can become a straight-jacket neither party would want to live with. For disagreements or interpretations over contract language or contract performance, fact-finding, mediation, or arbitration offer inexpensive, quick and peaceful alternatives. (These will be examined in chapter fifteen.)

Intent and Definition

With apparent agreement in hand, with all issues settled, the final step is to put it all in writing. Busy as you may be with your practice, try to be the one who will draft the memorandum of understanding that will be the basis for the signed agreement. Taking this initiative has several advantages: (1) The person who prepares the language of the basic agreement will usually take an inclusive interest in considering all the consequences of language interpretation; (2) Without changing the intent of agreement, clauses favorable to you can be written; and (3) By writing the agreement in your own words you can avoid legalisms and confusion.

In addition to the basic agreement which covers all areas that were discussed and confirmed, and in order to keep the basic agreement limited to the broader areas of understanding, you may need appendices to cover specific *intent* of clauses where such explanation may be necessary. Along with intent, there is the matter of definition of words or phrases that may have caused some confusion during the negotiation, especially where the words are susceptible to several meanings. Finally, appendices are a good place to include detailed procedures that are subject to change, as they can be updated without requiring renegotiation or change in the basic agreement.

If the negotiations were for an individual, and as that individual you are satisfied with the memorandum of understanding, sign it. If, on the other hand, you have been negotiating as the representative of a group or society your negotiating is not yet over because you have to get the approval of those you represented. Memorandum in hand, you now have to sell your settlement. As long as you have stayed within the guidelines given you by your peers, you should not have too difficult a job. If the negotiations have concluded with innovative solutions, a plan to sell the settlement should be prepared, because, unfortunately, those members who had nothing to do with the actual table talk and maneuvering of the negotiation have a tendency to try to impose the blue sky original wish-list against the final results to make the negotiator look less than efficient. So, preparation and temper control become necessary. This requirement too often turns out to be more trying and difficult than the negotiations recently concluded with an opponent. One problem is maintaining your opponent's credibility and trust when your principals send you back to the table to ask for additional concessions. Expect to be refused—and if your opponent is given a similar task, give him a firm "no." Both of you will recognize this ploy and send it back without further discussion. The other problem is maintaining the trust and credibility of your peers. Assure them that what you have accomplished is the very best that was possible at that time. If some points were not concluded to the group's satisfaction, point out that the agreement is for a limited period, and, if the group is still dissatisfied when the agreement runs out they can put those items back on the agenda with a better chance of success the second round.

When everyone is satisfied with the agreement language, the formal signing and effectuation can take place.

11

MAKING IT WORK

What we have done here is important . . . Too many have suffered . . . to throw it all away . . . We do not take proper care of what we have won with blood and sweat.

Alexander Kent,
Success to the Brave

With the drama successfully and satisfactorily concluded, the parties should not expect the agreement to work itself. Regardless of the friendly atmosphere in which the negotiations may have been conducted, the parties are adversaries. And, as with any adversarial relationship that is ongoing, the parties are committed to living together within the framework of an agreement. What has been created is the outline for administration of the agreement—at least for the duration of this agreement. What takes place in the administration of the agreement will, at least in part, establish the basis for the next negotiation or confrontation between the parties. It is one of the rules of thumb of the negotiation process that the time to begin preparation for the next negotiation is immediately after concluding the current agreement. Keep a file of all problems of interpretation and administration that arise in the course of the agreement, how they were handled, and who was responsible. This simplifies one's preparation for the next negotiation by having all the pertinent information in writing. In the crush of day-to-day professional practice it is difficult, without written record, to recall problems that took place months or years before.

Parties who negotiate an agreement are rarely the people who will administer it. The physician is in the same position as the legislators and general public after laws and ordinances are passed—the bureaucrats take over and administer those laws and ordinances according to their parochial views, prejudices, and presumptions. This overreaching can become a subtle brand of oppression. It becomes the task and responsibility of the signing parties to make sure that the administration of their agreement is done within the terms they understood and agreed to. *Any* movement away from the terms, intent or procedures confirmed by the signing must be immediately brought to the attention of the party that has begun to take license, and corrected. What may be the most critical attitude toward agreement administration is a clear appreciation of the rule that each party has the responsibility for the proper maintenance of his agreement. Neither party should ever be permitted the opportunity to impose his interpretation or change on the other, whether the change is frivolous or reasonable.

This admonition might seem overly simplistic, but do not ignore it. Agreements and contracts do not operate in a vacuum. If a clause is open to interpretation, someone who was not part of the negotiation process but is charged with its administration will always find words or clauses that require adaptation. This will create problems. Initiative for change, even if change should become necessary because of unforeseen developments, may come from either party but must be mutually agreed to or change cannot take place. What should be kept in mind is that administrators of the agreement particularly when they are non-negotiators, may and probably will take action where it is *not* prohibited by the language of the agreement. If such action takes place, and one of the parties believes that that action violates the intent or language of the agreement, he must immediately raise the issue with the other party to get either a correction or an understanding of how the administration of the agreement is to proceed. Be sure to have any changes written and signed by both parties, and retain a copy.

Making It Work

All this gives rise to a few guidelines for the handling of agreement interpretation and administration. Each party should remember the language that has resulted from the proposals, counterproposals, understandings, ideas withdrawn or turned down during the negotiations when confronted with an interpretive situation. (The possibility of arbitration is one of the important reasons for maintaining good notes during negotiations and not discarding them after the signing. One will be better prepared to meet the arbitrator with notes in hand.)

Items to be considered in administering an agreement:

- *Verbal or oral evidence:* Where the words of an agreement appear ambiguous, the parties' verbal recollection of their understanding at the time of agreement will be accepted. However, disagreement about the meaning of the language does not constitute ambiguity.
- *Memory vs. a Meeting of the Minds:* Too often, we assume the meanings of words as they have been understood in the light of our own experience. If we did not, at the time an issue was discussed and settled, question an opponent as to his understanding, the written language can be ambiguous. At such times, depending upon the submission limitations placed upon the third party, arbitrators will not substitute their judgment for the specific language at issue. (Most arbitration clauses specifically deny the arbitrator the flexibility to modify agreement language by adding to or subtracting from the written agreement.)
- *Intent vs. Law:* In cases where there are definite but alternative interpretations of the written agreement, the choice or decision must adhere to the law because the assumption is made that neither party intentionally intended to contravert the law.
- *Word Usage:* When neither party can reasonably establish interpretation of ambiguous words, those words will usually be taken in their popularly accepted meaning. (Basic to this assumption is the acceptance of the theory that the parties were negotiating honestly and in good faith with each other and had all good intentions of working out a sound agreement. However, "popularly accepted meaning" could, when down to the nitty-gritty, turn out to be a third meaning.) Should the words involved be terms peculiar to medical or health care, they will be viewed in the professional context unless the apparent intent of the totality suggests differently.
- *Consistency—of Words, Context, Total Agreement:* In any controversy over meaning and intent, words will be interpreted in the context of others used: Words or phrases will be viewed for the way they also give significance to other parts of the agreement, so that dissimilar interpretations do not create further interpretive conflicts. Words will be assumed to have the same meaning throughout the total agreement, unless in the section in dispute they were specifically defined in another way.
- *Precedent and Past Practice:* Both precedent and past practice can indicate intent. This type of word usage usually results from past

failures to object to the handling of situations covered by the agreement over an extended period. Questions can be raised as to whether or not the injured party had been notified of the change, or should have been aware of what was being done. The aggrieved party has to establish a *de minimus* situation, one or at most only a few alleged misinterpretations to deny precedent establishment, or show that the words or clause are truly unambiguous. However, if an unobjected word or clause is allowed to be carried over into subsequent agreements, it will be assumed that both parties knew and agreed to the practice. On the other hand, if the aggrieved party can demonstrate a general acceptance or usage of his position or interpretation among his peers, his view may prevail.

- *Drafting Intent:* As noted earlier, it is advisable for a negotiator to draft the final agreement. When taking on such a task, one must try not to have too many potentially ambiguous words, although it is the task of the other party to review what has been written. While the courts tend to hold ambiguities against the agreement writer, jointly reviewed agreements can be presumed to have been arrived at equally. This is an area of negotiation where, if both parties leave the work to others, such as lawyers, where language peculiar to that trade rather than to the health professionals may be used, ambiguity can arise.

What is at stake in the administration of your agreement is all the work that was put into getting it. Carelessness or inattention to how your rights and rewards under an agreement are provided for can waste the time and effort you put into reaching the agreement. Permitting the establishment of a precedent or undesirable practice cannot be blamed on anyone but the party that allowed it to happen. Should the other party to your agreement manage to alter the intent of any part of your agreement without prior notice, and over time manages to maintain that change without objection on your part, he will always be prepared to say "But you haven't objected so far. Why now?" The time to question is the moment that you recognize any deviation from the agreement. For the individual concerned with his own agreement, there should be no problem; all he has to do is talk to his opposite signer. If that doesn't correct the situation, he has the due process section of the agreement to fall back on for correction. For a group, the problem becomes one of internal communication. One person should be responsible for handling aspects of agreement relationships with the other party to the agreement. All members of the group should funnel complaints, information about bureaucratic tinkering with the intent of their agreement, or any other inconsistencies to that person. (This is the person who should be keeping the log for the next negotiations.) This requires that everyone in the group be knowledgeable, first, of the agreement and what it is meant to accomplish, and second, of the need for each member who learns of the other party's tinkering to immediately notify the group's intermediary.

Successfully concluding negotiations with a satisfactory win/win result is important but no more so than making it work in practice. This is gospel; don't ignore it. Negotiation, often described as an "art," should not create sand castles that will be washed away with the tide. If you have negotiated a solid agreement, be ready for someone to start chipping away, a little at a time. Be ready, not to depend upon goodwill alone, but upon the practical application of all that you worked for. Vigilance and prompt response to unwanted tinkering is the only answer to arbitrary opponent action and will make all the effort and time that you put into your negotiations worthwhile.

12

PROTECTIVE ORGANIZATION—DOCTORS AND UNIONS

Only organize, and stand together. Claim something together, and at once; let the nation hear a united demand from the laboring voice, and then, when you have got that, go on after another; but get something.

Wendell Phillips, 1870

Faced with the pressures of increasing regulatory restrictions and anticipating an oversupply of physicians, hospitals and other health service functions are expanding their staffs of employee-physicians. Where once the members of a hospital staff enjoyed a recognized position in the hospital administration pecking order, that role has been brought down several pegs by professional pursuit outside the hospital and malpractice suits within the hospital. Today, administrators, as the representatives of boards of directors, dominate health care services hierarchies. The employed physician trained to practice as an independent, tends to take a disinterested and somewhat disdainful view of employee organizing.

As suggested earlier, the members of the hospital medical staff unquestionably have suffered in recent years some reduction of status within the hospital. The independent fee-for-service physician is better off in terms of status. He or she is really a customer of the hospital who brings patients to it for care that is not readily available in the office or the patient's home. They can work at arm's length with hospital administration.

Not so employed physicians. They are subject to the vagaries of hospital politics and do not enjoy the leverage of the free-standing physician. Like most physicians, the employed doctor seems to have a built-in aversion to employee organizing.

The foundation for employee-physician organization has been academically stated by John A. Buesseler, M.D., M.S., as Buesseler's Socioeconomic Law: "Oligopsony Begets Oligopoly" meaning that "As a large number of buyers collectivize into a small number of organized buyers, the large number of sellers will defensively collectivize into a small number of sellers."

Buesseler's Law can be updated or rephrased to indicate that, as hospitals become larger and their administrations become more secure and powerful through favorable legal interpretation or as smaller hospitals combine their purchasing to distribute savings for common services, growing numbers of physicians hired by those hospitals will find it to their mutual good to organize within those employer units in self-defense. Any effort in this direction will be not to control (defined in *Webster* as "to exercise restraining or directing influence over; regulate) but to gain and retain a fairer status with the employers.

Why Organize?

Because the focus of medical education and training is extremely conservative, it produces physicians who are unattracted to the idea of protective organization (unionization). This attitude becomes self-perpetuating because their professional pride and the information available to them do not permit them to look beyond the facade of media accounts of industrial and hospital unions' strife. Ultimately the best guarantee of decent working conditions and the end to the various excessive patterns of bureaucratic discrimination is an employee organization agreement (contract). Such an agreement, written around the concerns of locally employed physicians, gives them the legal framework within which subsequent renegotiations or other issues can be discussed and settled. Without the protection of a written agreement employed physicians will continue to be vulnerable, fragmented, and critically impotent as they deal with employers to secure the full professional benefits for which they work. Combined with their employee peers they will secure what the unorganized professionals sorely lack, a single voice with which to shape and state their views and protect their jobs. The steps taken toward professional organization will depend upon how well the physicians can articulate, how well their elected leadership can translate understanding of the memberships' needs and work-related issues.

Organizing employee-physicians would seem to have at least three strikes for a person having such an interest: a lack of cooperative consciousness; the lack of viable physician organization examples; and groups of individuals with no history or experience of organizing. Professionalism hangs like an albatross from their necks, dividing them, and separating them into limited classifications. Against this Lone Ranger mentality organization development has a tremendous job even to get employee-physicians to understand that they cannot solve all their problems as individuals. However, when faced with (1) an increasing bureaucratization of their working environment, (2) the progressive dichotomy between fee-for-service professionals and employed physicians, and, eventually, (3) their perceived need to avoid crises at work that are apparently created by opponents whose own selfish interests are basically vested in opposition, employed physicians may be able to be convinced of the need to organize.

Smooth, trained administration representatives, intent upon maintaining a union-free organization that they can control either through intimidation or dissuasion, will have a pat response when faced with an employed physician who raises questions about working conditions: "There's the door. If you don't like the way we do things here, you can leave." Most doors, as we learn early in life, swing two ways. And that is where an organized occupational group can become effective in protecting and enhancing its science and perquisites. What is needed is a composite but single voice with a contract to protect the membership both as a group and as individuals. That protection can only be had through a cover organization. With that, problems can be worked out, without having a Damoclean sword of termination without due process hanging over each employed physician's head.

Employee-physician organizations will develop because their members are faced with issues of mutual concern. The development of an active professional employee-group with a series of unresolved issues offers both parties opportunities to meet under mutually acceptable conditions to discuss and resolve those issues with their employers, and to avoid open controversy. Some of the issues or problems that could be better handled by group representation include: security, staffing (and its implications of speedup with a concomitant loss of professional integrity), safety (both for the physicians and the hospital employees and patients), supervision (as practiced by the administration's bureaucracy, and as required of the physicians), stress, scheduling, professional respect and dignity, due process and continuing educational opportunities. Included with these general problems would, of course, be any strictly local issues. This localized problem-solving approach for employed physicians is seriously and enthusiastically recommended. With the added protection of the National Labor Relations Act, the local approach is the most desirable and legitimate method in which to engage.

A *caveat* is in order for physicians employed by public (city, county, state, federal) bodies. As more states accept the principle of public employee organization, the makeup of the employee representative groups becomes most important. To limit the number of contracts that need to be negotiated and administered, public bodies will attempt to include all types of "professionals" into a large group. This can be disastrous for physicians. As a minority within a designated bargaining unit, physicians will be voted into obscurity by other factions of the unit. Physicians should make every attempt to remain a separate and independent unit or they will be forced to take on the actions (strikes, work actions, etc.) of the unit majority.

Getting the Act Together

Employed physician organizing usually begins with discussions between troubled individuals who, because of leadership potential or recognized influence within the employed group, are able to express and translate ideas into statements that relate to specific professional-employer problems. Articulate and respected physicians within the group are helpful to the organizing process.

Depending upon the number of physicians and the specialties that may or can be included for representation to the employer, leadership should be limited to a single person from each component. The problem at this stage of organization is to maintain secrecy as long as possible to surprise the employer when the group asks for recognition. Premature notice of the effort will quickly result in a maximum "divide and conquer" drive by the administration. Such a drive includes, at the least: firings, offers of individualized increases and other perks, and much personalized attention. In the long run, however, all the buddy-buddy cosmetics will fade and conditions will revert to the way they were. Should this happen, every effort must be made to keep the group together, with each member disclosing completely all advances and propositions offered by the administration.

Depending upon the size of the group to be organized, alternative approaches are available. First, for the small group—the professional staff of a pathology lab or a radiology section, the organizing can eliminate most of the actions to be taken for a large group such as the professional staff of an HMO. A small group, after feelers reveal a number of frustrations and problems, can get together to pool their differences with an administration to develop a comprehensive program. Along with this pooling of grievances, the group should review the major policies and practices of the administration as they apply to the group, and bring out the differences between policy, as written, and practice, as it differs from the stated policy. Meetings of the group should *not* be held on the premises. No point in letting the administration know what is going on until everything is ready to be put into effect.

In a larger group, once the leaders have found each other and have banded together, their first order of business should be the pooling of their frustrations and grievances. They should work up a comprehensive picture of the physician group. A secretary should be appointed or elected who will maintain the *only* written records for the organizing period. A preliminary review of the employer's policies and practices that may be responsible for general discontent of the employed physicians should be included in the early meetings. Most important at this time is the organization of an information network that will be extremely helpful in keeping tabs on what the employer administration is currently doing.

For the core group to begin its work on a solid foundation, information about the total employed physician in their group should include:

- the departmental or specialty structure of the organization;
- the number of physicians in each department or specialty, by shift or by other appropriate designation;
- estimates of departmental morale, reactions to local rules and procedures;
- physicians who may be considered leaders in their departments—these will be the early contacts to be made by the core group;
- administration methods of communicating with employee-physicians for handling their problems and gripes; and,
- benefits and perks, overall and by department.

Questions that will elicit the information desired, while maintaining the secrecy needed at this stage of organizing, might include:

- "Since joining our organization, what work-related incident or incidents have negatively affected your practice-behavior?"
- "What incident(s) had greater impact than others on your attitude or feelings toward working as an employee in contrast to your attitudes or feelings before joining our organization?"
- "Tell me about this incident(s)—the setting, its duration."
- "What person or persons were involved in this incident(s) and what

effect did that person or persons have on the event(s)? What effect did it have on others who may have been witness?''

- ''What were your personal reactions to the incident(s)?''
- ''What are your feelings about practicing medicine as an employee today as compared to your impressions or expectations when you completed your training or when you first planned to become a physician?''

When developing their basic organization, the core group will be concerned primarily with the quality rather than the quantity of their contacts. Because the nitty-gritty job of group development will probably take place in open meeting places—corridors, coffee rooms, etc.—the primary goal of bringing people together for the common cause can best begin by a relatively small core.

Internal Communication

At this stage of the organization the core group should have developed a working plan for its internal communication. Addresses, telephone numbers, beeper designations, working schedules, and other personal data that would be necessary to enable them to contact each other quickly should be exchanged. Since telephone communication can be the fastest means of contacting the organizers' growing number of supporters, a pyramid chart listing telephone and beeper designations, described below, is most effective. As each member in the chain of communication completes his calls, he reports the results to his senior in the chain of organization.

Along with the development of the communications network, a funding base must be developed. Some funds will become needed for pamphlets, letters, and social contacts. Funds required will not be exorbitant, but with the knowledge that each has made a financial investment, the new and latecomers to the organization have a more personal interest in seeing the organizing succeed.

There is no set rule for the core group's next step. They may decide to begin their campaign to acquire employee-physician signatures authorizing a ''Germinal ____________ Physicians' Association'' to represent them in meetings with the employer organization. This can be accomplished either through petitions or signed cards. Whatever the means, each physician should be approached for his signature and financial commitment authorizing the core group to ''. . . develop an Association to represent the physicians of the *(employer)*.'' A card similar to what follows should be signed by all potential members:

> To Whom It May Concern:
>
> I authorize the ______________ Physicians' Coordinating Committee to develop an Association of employed physicians to represent me and the physician staff of said employer.
>
> ______________________
> (signature)
>
> ______________
> (date)
>
> (CONFIDENTIAL)

At this stage the physicians are only being asked to back the organizing effort with their signatures and a small contribution. They must be assured that the cards or petitions will be kept confidential and together in one safe place. Signatures alone should not be considered a positive commitment to the core group's effort. However, having signed the authorization and probably having made some small financial contribution, they will have an interest in the association's development, and, as organizing continues, efforts will be made to get each signer more intimately involved in the campaign.

To avoid duplication of card-signing efforts, the core group should develop and maintain contact charts in an accessible but confidential location for the purposes of organization, enlistment, and communication flow. An organization chart may look something like the one that follows.

What develops here is known as the "nucleus" tactic of organizing. It is the cell approach in which, at successive levels of the organization, each person, after being integrated into the ideas and purposes of the organization, goes out to recruit and integrate several others. The size of the potential membership and the number in the core group will determine the number of levels on the organization chart. One caveat to be observed at this stage of organization and recruitment is as much secrecy as possible. Brown will work with only A and B; A will only know Brown, Smith and Gray as members; and so on. The nuclei cells should be listed only on the records of the core group secretary. Along with the organization chart, it becomes advisable to have rosters of all physicians who are potential members, set up both by department or specialty service and alphabetically. With this combination of charts and rosters the core group can maintain an up-to-date listing of enlisted and as yet uncommitted or unsolicited members. They will also prevent the wasteful duplication of effort in organizing.

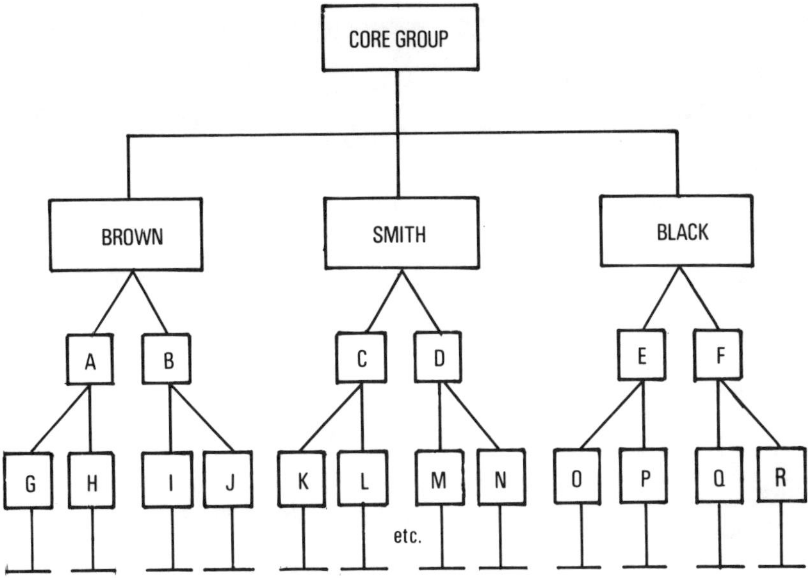

(with each name, department & telephone no.)

Campaigning and Participation: Maintaining Momentum

The campaign hangs on the framework of issues and concerns. There may be situations for which no immediate or obvious issues exist. Such situations, few and far between as they may be, do *not* automatically preclude developing an employed-physician organization. A recognized group will be able to recommend improvements, alert administrations to potential problems, and negotiate on behalf of the employee group, avoiding conflict and potential morale problems.

Back to the issues and the campaign to unify the physicians. Fellow employees have been recruited, cards have been signed, and a small war chest has been built. Participation, both passive (most members will back the purposes of the group but, by nature and the residual effects of resident training, will prefer to remain in the background) and active with continuing interest in the organization, must be maintained. It is difficult to get and keep full attendance at meetings on any kind of regular basis because of work schedules, so personal contacts, letters, and pamphlets will have to

DEPARTMENT ROSTER

Family Practice	card signed	fees paid
A	x	x
B.	x	
C.		
D.	x	x
E.		
F.	x	x
G.	x	
Internal medicine		
H.	x	x
I	x	
J.	x	x
K.	x	x
Surgery		
L.		
M		
N	x	x
O.		

etc.

ALPHABETICAL ROSTER

A	x	x
B.	x	
C.		
D.	x	x
E.		
F.	x	x
G.	x	
H.	x	x
I	x	

etc.

be the primary method for disseminating information. Communications from the core group must be kept short, clear, and specifically to the issues and organizing progress. *The most effective technique is the personal one-on-one conversation.*

If the group to be organized is, beside being fairly large, difficult to congregate at one time because of schedules, locations, and administrative functions, communications may have to take the pamphlet route. Also, if the core group, in reaching out for additional supporters finds that its vocal abilities are not as convincing as its ideas and need for organization, written solicitations may be more effective. The first publication should state, concisely, but in general terms, the reasons for organizing. Subsequent publications and the frequency of their distribution will gradually become more specific.

After becoming acquainted with the overall rationale for organizing, the employed physicians will begin asking "What's in it for me?" and "How will this affect me in my job?" As the campaign develops, communications will deal with specific issues, relations with the administration, and with the association's program. The frequency of letters or pamphlets will depend upon the type of campaign, the number of potential members, the use and effectiveness of various forms of communication, reactions of the administration, and the leaders' assessments of the group's needs. As the campaign peaks, frequency of publication will increase to a more regular schedule. Each printed piece (mimeographed, photocopied, etc.) should meet three criteria: (1) it must have eye-appeal to encourage the physician to read it; (2) it must present only one, two, or at the very most, three issues in precise and concise language; and (3) it must suggest credible and preferably non-inflammatory means for dealing with the issue(s).

The most attractive printed pieces present the maximum possible white space. Eyes are prone to be lazy or tired—especially after reading medical books and journals. Single-spaced pages look too busy, appear too difficult to read. When possible, use humorous items clipped from newspapers and magazines, that emphasize the particular issue. A headline, traced with the help of a lettering guide, creates interest by summarizing or highlighting the message. Keep sentences and paragraphs short, and use simple words. Adopt the basic journalistic practice of putting key information in the first and second paragraphs—the rest of the piece fills in the details. Again, remember to leave plenty of white space and try to keep the whole message on one side of the sheet, using fourteen-inch paper if necessary. Finally, each paper should have the name of the organization prominently displayed and should be signed, either by the whole coordinating core group or by several of its members, one or two at a time.

Consider mailing leaflets to the physician's home. This serves a dual purpose. You'll get the message to the physician when he has time to read and think about it. It also gets the message to the spouses, keeps them informed about what is going on at their spouses' workplace, and can serve as an additional inducement for reluctant physicians to join their peers.

Organization and Commitment

Keep the membership and the hesitants informed. This is what is behind the cliché "getting it together"—even though the thinking members will appreciate that the issues and goals are basically relative and subject to change. It is good to understand that, as Saul Alinsky has pointed out, the "establishment in many ways is as suicidal as (those who call themselves radical), except that they are infinitely more inclined to be self-destructive than those radicals will ever be." Lacking open communication, the members will remain effectively silent and inactive. Unfortunately, silence and avoidance of commitment will be assumed and promoted by an administration as acquiescence to their status quo. A knowledgeable group will coalesce and support its leaders. Questions must be answered so that the unity of the group can be maintained. Diplomacy is essential in organizing situations, so only as much information as is necessary to maintain interest should be provided. Issues are the key. The more articulately the issues can be stated—quality patient care, services both to the patients and the administration, community services, potential cost-savings, absence of due process, etc.—the better the organizing effort will be.

Regardless of the issues and their importance to the well-being of the employed group in total, physicians tend to be an impatient lot. They tend to become bored with the preliminaries that are essential to purposeful action. Effective pursuit of organization gains may be frustrated by the desire for quick and dramatic change. Among the cautions that the core group must teach their potential membership: achievement of recognition and an eventual agreement will take time. They must understand that seldom does anyone *like* to move away from the mental security of what has become familiar to them, and that the apparent leisurely pace of organizing provides a sort of bridge to get them to a new way of practice and away from their present system that has proven self-deprecating and frustrating. It is not easy to "keep the heat on" an administration, but that is where the action will come from.

In this phase of organizing you want commitment. As noted, one of the best ways to ensure that commitment is through individual contributions to the coordinating committee's treasury. Besides money, commitment can also take the form of personal investments of time and service—hence the organizing pyramid. Financial and/or personal involvement begets loyalty to the cause.

Some flexibility is required at this stage in order to determine the issues and potential solutions that are most important to the membership. Issues, once delineated, should be reiterated. The goal is to receive positive and committed answers from the administration. The association as an ongoing unit performs this service.

Achieving Recognition

Formal and legal recognition of the association of employed physicians is the goal of organizing. The best way to get this recognition is with the assistance of the National Labor Relations Board (NLRB). Once the NLRB is brought into the picture, legal safeguards take effect, foreclosing, in most instances, retributive actions by the administration. Going to the board for help in having a formal election to certify your association can be the first step. This action can help members of an employed physician group realize how they may be taken advantage of by an entrenched administration. To vent one's frustrations, especially in a perfectly legal manner, is an achievement in creative justice. And this kind of achievement becomes sweeter against what, in many cases, have become bottom-line operations run by largely unimaginative, staid and sometimes insensitive people. (Somehow, corporate employees often become self-centered bureaucrats soon after rising within a corporation, putting aside their creativity and ego-identity for the security of the corporate womb.)

Once the group has become viable it probably has become known to the administration. The core group should notify the administration, in writing, that the organization exists and that it is prepared to meet with the employer to discuss mutual problems, represented by Drs. _____, _____, etc. Disclosure of the leaders' names prevents the administration from any precipitate action against those leaders under the board rules. (This does not rule out underhanded attempts to "get back" at the leaders through allegations of failure to follow administrative procedures which, of course, from this point on everyone must be sure to observe to the letter.) In many cases the administration will refuse to recognize the association either on the word of the leaders that they represent the will of the employed physicians, or upon presentation of a petition signed by most of the doctors, and insist upon dawdling through the process of having a formal NLRB or state election. Petitions should be worded along the lines of: "The undersigned recognize the _____ Physicians' Association as their official representative and delegate to it the power and authority to represent us in discussions and agreements in matters of patient care, hours, salaries, benefits, and related matters."

In those cases where the physicians are employed by public hospitals or other public health institutions, there may be a state public employee law that authorizes public employee collective bargaining. After consultation with and upon the advice of qualified local counsel, physicians may be able to utilize their local laws to achieve recognition. Do not work with any attorney in any way associated with a public or private healthcare administration. An industrial labor lawyer can offer the best assistance at this stage of the organizing.

If local laws are either unavailable or are advised against by counsel, bring the NLRB into the picture. The board will authorize what is called a "Representation Election" when shown that thirty percent of the employees have signed the petition for recognition. Following hearings to determine the scope and duties of the employee group (which the administration counsel may try to extend and disrupt) the board will set a mutually satisfactory date for an election that will be conducted by a board representative by secret ballot. (Although the board will go ahead with an election on the basis of a thirty percent petition, it is advisable that the core group have not less than sixty or seventy per cent of the employed physicians signed up. Even better would be to have the signatures of *all* members of the group as a positive commitment.) If the election confirms that fifty per cent plus one of those voting are in favor of the association's stated desires, the association becomes the authorized representative bargaining agent for the physicians and the employer must recognize the association, under penalty of law.

Recognition elections are lost as often as they are won. Members forget to vote, misunderstand the need to vote (A "no show" is, effectively, the same as a "No" vote), or, for some inexplicable reason, simply disappear into the woodwork. If there are any detractors who have been suborned by the administration, they will be busy spreading innuendoes, misinformation and outright lies. (Once an election has been set, clarification of all rumors, questions and anti-physician association comments should be funnelled to a "truth squad" for clarification and exposition.)

The newsletter, and verbal communication through the organization pyramid, should emphasize patient care deficiencies and administrative shortcomings as the more important issues before the group, while maintaining contact with the issues that brought the group into being. In going after victory in an election for recognition, the administration may unwittingly become your best advocate because it tends to overstate and make irrational assertions. As long as you do not panic by trying to answer their charges, these exaggerations will tend to be treated as jokes. Overbearing tactics are neither in good taste or effective. The newsletter should be informative, stressing the routine nature of the election process and the unassailable fact that it is sanctioned by the U.S. Government, and being resorted to more and more by professionals. The most vital information that stands repetition in winning an election is that on the day set for the vote, *all* supporters of the association *must* get to the polling place *and vote*. Use the verbal contacts of your organization pyramid to inform any association detractors how their actions are truly self-defeating for the general welfare of all employed physicians—but be sure that acrimony, debate, and general pushiness or ''coventry'' tactics are avoided.

Again, avoid mud-slinging contests with the administration. Remember that after the election and the drawn-out negotiations that will undoubtedly ensue, you and all the members of the association will have to coexist. Any basis for ongoing bad feelings will only make for a poor and unproductive working relationship. Stress the positive reasons for the association activities, the goals being sought, and how all will benefit, not only the physicians but the patients and the community as well. If throughout the election campaign your newsletter and other communications have informed the membership and moderated the fears of the vacillating, and group members work to get every available and potential voter to the polls, the group should be assured of victory.

With certification and recognition in hand, negotiation meetings become the order of the day. Goal-setting, preparation, the drama, and agreement have all been covered earlier. Ratification will require the same kind of effort that went into organizing and negotiating. Because expectations will almost always be more optimistic than the final results of negotiations that pragmatic and flexible handling dictated, the members may have to be ''sold'' that the agreement is the best that could be negotiated at *this* time, that there will be more agreements to negotiate, and that each member has responsibility for making this work.

Successful organization doesn't happen, it requires determination, humor and, often, a thick skin. For employed physicians, the effort is worth the goal.

An Organizing Philosophy

No one in the Twentieth Century has personified and achieved the causes of consumer activist groups better than Saul Alinsky. This community organizer developed innovative tactics to create the image of power to get results. In his book, *Rules for Radicals,* Alinsky sets guidelines that help organize employed physicians. The following ideas can be transferred to employed-physician use and applied to their process of organizing and beyond:

- **Power is not just what you possess, but what your opponent believes you possess and use.** As long as physicians retain the goodwill of their patients and do nothing to disrupt that relationship, hospitals and insurors (private and government) will have to tread with some caution in any proceedings against physicians, either as individuals or as a profession. Physicians, working with and through their patients (the hospitals' and insurors' clients) to exercise and express their favorable views of the physicians, create a *perception* of "physician power" to those hospitals and insurors.

- **Keep your tactics within the experience of your supporters.** Using the physician/patient relationship as the base for confrontation, the exercise of a little more human relations within those relationships can greatly aid development of the perception projected above. If actions or tactics are outside the day-to-day experiences of your supporters, confusion, anxiety and a collapse of communications can result.

- **Whenever possible, direct your arguments to ideas and presumptions that are outside your opponents' experience.** Hospitals and insurors often take the attitude that they are benefactors to their clients. Confuse them and compound their perception of "physician power" by insisting that they are only purveyors of purchased services whose clients are demanding all that has been purchased.

- **Make an opponent live up to the rules he claims to live by.** When an opponent insists that he is "going by the book", insist on seeing the book, question the authority for what is written. For example, rules published in the Federal Register by government agencies can have the force of law as long as they do not subvert or misdirect the intent of the authorizing legislation. However, the bureaucracies often issue innumerable explanations and interpretations that eventually create contradictions; these are always kept within the issuing service and are not published, thus being of questionable value as against the rule or the law. You will also find that that opponent hasn't read the book lately, depending on others to tell him the department's interpretation as verbalized through a variety of previous interpreters. Left unchallenged, those interpretations develop precedential bases that may be difficult to overturn. Go up the bureaucratic ladder for clarifications and confusions, and insist on their adherence to their rules—especially if that favors your position—and public apology by publication of the correct method, etc., to the served public. You can fight City Hall, if only to a draw.

- **Ridicule can be one of your most effective weapons.** It is almost impossible to counterattack ridicule. It will usually infuriate the opponent and cause him to react in a manner that will be to your advantage.
- **Good tactics are those that your own people enjoy being part of.** Particularly when you are working with a group of physicians, anything that can be included to pep up the development of an organization or ease the tediousness of an extended negotiation to maintain both interest and enjoyed concern is a good tactic.
- **Any tactic that becomes a drag has gone on too long.** The whole process of organization is built around the strategy of putting and keeping pressure upon the employer. Interest can be maintained in a project for a reasonable but limited time if it remains only a verbal commitment. This means that a succession of tactical maneuvers must be prepared to rejuvenate your group's interest when it begins to flag. Given the proper and varied applications of pressures, an opponent will eventually react, which can lead to some tactical error which, if promptly advantaged should improve your negotiating stance.
- **A perceived threat is usually more frightening than either the actual threat or the act of carrying it through.** Imagination is often your best weapon. The implication that patients will not receive care, that selected rules of an organization will be observed either in the breach or not at all, can be more effective than the actual action. Take care though; you're not playing in a poker game. *If you aren't ready and able to carry it out successfully, don't bluff or threaten.* If your opponent catches you in a bluff and calls it, your credibility suffers and future threats will be downgraded or ignored.

- **Any negative approach of an opponent confronted hard and deep enough will result eventually in a positive action.** Pointing loudly and often at an opponent's high-handed—or underhanded—actions with outraged alarm, shock, and moral injury may be used to force positive reactions to a negative position taken by that opponent. This can be part of the pressure constant.
- **Don't rest on your laurels just because a tactic succeeds; have another one ready.** A successful opponent tactic is to agree occasionally outright with a demand. Don't let up at that victory. Be prepared with followup and increasing pressures. For example, faced with "We don't know what to do about the situation you describe; who does?" you had better have alternate solutions that further your goals ready.
- **A corporation or agency is difficult to target. Pick a person-target, immobilize him as the target, personalize and polarize that target.** Because most of the targets of an organizing campaign are usually generalized subjects, interesting because of the ramifications of their effects on the employee population, they do not have personality. By personalizing an opponent in terms that both your group and the public can understand—"Administrator Jones expects us to _____ _____, and won't even discuss why or how with us!"—you can change the focus of attention from issues to personality, bring an element of fun to the situation, and acquire allies who may previously have been unwilling to openly support your goals. The only caveat that should be observed in personalizing a situation is not to get vicious—after the dust settles, you will have to live with the object of that personalizing, and he will still be the boss.

How can these tactics be applied to organization and negotiations by physicians? They represent much of what others are doing to them as a class; properly positioned to reverse the others' attacks, they can be an excellent base for an effective offense.

A *verbum sapienti* for everyone who sees the need and begins to organize and/or to represent physicians might well be in order in closing this section by quoting Isaiah (VI, 9–10):

> "And He said, Go, and say unto this people, Hear indeed, but understand not; and see indeed, but know not.
>
> Obdurate will remain the heart of this people, and their ears will be heavy, and their eyes will be shut; so that they will not see with their eyes, nor hear with their ears, nor their hearts be understanding, so that they be converted, and healing granted them."

How better to describe healthcare bureaucrats?

13

CONTRACTS—LEGAL LABYRINTHS OR THE BASE OF A WORKING RELATIONSHIP

I have found that to make a contented slave it is necessary to make a thoughtless one. It is necessary to darken his mental and moral vision, and, as far as possible, to annihilate the power of reason. He must be able to detect no inconsistencies in slavery; he must be made to feel that slavery is right; and he can be brought to that only when he ceases to be a man.

Frederick Douglass, 1845

Contracts, whether formal or informal agreements between providers of medical care and support, are more prevalent in the healthcare field than many of us imagine. The latest published study of the American Medical Association (1981) reports that approximately 78,600 (out of 485,123) non-federal[1] physicians practice under some form of contract. These figures may not include contracts between physicians as employees or independent contractors with government agencies, teaching institutions, HMO's, or other forms of non-hospital health service functions.

A contract can be a written or unwritten agreement between parties. It is usually for a definite term and it defines the conditions under which the parties will fulfill their obligations to each other. The rights and responsibilities of the parties, and the procedures to be followed in settling contract disputes or handling previously unexpected problems that may arise during the term of the agreement should also be included. The need for written agreements between consenting parties is becoming more important as hospitals and other healthcare organizations become more conscious of the responsibilities being placed on them by the major insur-

[1]If you include residents and federal physicians, the total with hospital and other contractual arrangements goes well over 156,000.

ors of healthcare and by the courts. Further complicating the necessity for clear and explicit agreements between physicians and health-oriented organizations—and, in most cases, negating the use of "boilerplate" or "model" contracts—are such concerns as the limitations imposed by organization bylaws and the authority of negotiators of contracting agents to bind their principals to performance. Physician contracts should be based upon and written to establish credible working relationships that will provide quality health care.

Components of a Good Contract

The successful contract will seek to achieve these goals: clear and positive language that will avoid misunderstandings; establishment of working relationships and ethical medical practices; assurance of the opportunities to work with minimal direct supervisory interference; methods and progression of payments; specifics of liabilities; including exclusivity within a specialty; clear and meaningful communication; termination only for proper cause; and due process free of bias. Contracts that satisfy these goals will assure *both* parties that there will be favorable and supportive working relationships. The reasoning behind these goal requirements include:

- *Avoiding misunderstandings.* Most misunderstandings are the result of *assumptions.* Where there may be some doubts during the negotiation of a contract, most physicians tend to avoid clearing up those doubts by asking for a full explanation for fear of appearing less than knowledgeable about the subject, and *assume* the opponent's meaning. Because, too often, the assumptions are at variance with the physician's intent, trouble between the parties will eventually surface. To avoid potential misunderstandings, spell out your intentions and question the other person's words—especially the apparently obvious ones.
- *Working relationships and ethical medical practices.* Having to work in conformity with a detailed job description can become enervating to the practice of one's specialty. The freedom and flexibility of judgment that are required to exercise one's training and experience can be hampered under such constraints. Also, there may be times when the bottom-line mentality of a commercially oriented organization will either suggest or insist that actions contrary to medical ethics be taken. Specificity is all right for enumerating the duties and responsibilities

of the other signer to a contract; good if you can tie him down. However, the physician's duties and responsibilities should be kept as broad as possible. If the other party insists that certain specifics be agreed to, put them in a side memorandum, using such words as "oversee," "direct," "show concern for," etc. Usually, by being specific and up front about the way you want to practice within the framework of a contract, you may be able to avoid many constraints.

- *Payments.* Methods and progression of payments will vary according to the status of the physician as employee or as consultant ("independent contractor"). If an employee, remuneration should be specified as to amount and period covered, benefits (insurances, vacations, hours, pensions, etc.) as well as regularity of reviews. If a consultant, remuneration either in monies or in support for research or practice using the other's facilities, should be spelled out.
- *Communication.* In most cases, there will probably be progress reports required on a regular basis. Records should be available without restraint so that each party works with the other with full knowledge of what is going on. Apart from the formal communication of reports and meetings, each should understand that the other can be approached for verbal communication whenever questions or problems develop. (While something like this is difficult to phrase in contract terms, it must be made clear to each other so that the relationship works without the development of petty distrusts.)
- *Termination. Due process.* Unfortunately, the trend, particularly for employed physicians, is for employer organizations to seek termination clauses that require only notice. In the forseeable future, with competition in the larger metropolitan areas increasing for the available medical positions, having such a clause in a contract—albeit the clause will read that *either* party may sever the relationship on so many days' notice—offers the employer the opportunity to hire a less expensive but more hungry physician with no organization responsibility to the present jobholder. A strong effort to add some variation of the phrase ". . . for proper (or sufficient/just) cause" to any termination clause will provide some protection. "Cause" is, of course, subject to legal interpretation, but generally is accepted as being an act of gross misbehavior or moral turpitude. Another phrase or idea that can make an employer think twice before summarily cutting the umbilical cord of employment would be one that will require the em-

ployer to pay through the end of the contract in case of termination for any or no reason other than proper cause. What you are after is some form of protection from an arbitrary action on the part of the other party to a contract. Should you be unable to get either of the above into your new agreement, hold out for not less than any termination of contract being subject to the medical staff bylaws, a much weaker assist than the others but at least some protection. Everyone, even administrators, will talk as though they are in favor of progress as long as it doesn't result in a change of their prerogatives. And prerogatives are at issue here; the prerogatives of management to plan, hire and *fire* that have perpetuated the adversary aspects of industrial labor/management relations.

A restrictive covenant may be included as an adjunct to termination. A contracting hospital, group, or employer may want a promise that the other party will refrain from providing specific services within a specific area for some extended time period following termination. To be legally enforceable, such covenant must be reasonable in both duration and scope. The reason for the restriction is to prevent competition. Some states either prohibit or limit restrictive covenants. If damages are related to the financial loss a party may suffer on account of the termination, they may be legally enforceable.

Negotiating contracts with a healthcare provider, particularly exclusive ones, can pose difficult issues for both parties. Because an increasing number of specialties and sub-specialties are becoming hospital-based, their practitioners are more involved with the hospitals' providing increased and more comprehensive services, inside and beyond the institution complex. The growth of health centers requires responsibilities for both hospitals and the physicians utilizing those extended services of more than just medical staff membership. As the hospitals' services increase, their bylaws change, making the writing of new or renegotiated agreements subject to those changes. Where the new hospital policies infringe on traditional physician prerogatives, care must be taken with the required new language to maintain the integrity of medical practice. *All* new or renegotiated contracts should be reviewed by all the medical contractors in order to maintain an equilibrium within the medical staff. If a general collaboration is not achieved among the physicians, the hospital—or any healthcare group—will be in the position of being able to manipulate the contracting physicians.

Contracts written by lawyers can be legal labyrinths. They can mean the difference between an agreement that you thought was good for your future and something that can be costly in time, money, and professional standing. Even more offensive, when you have to live with and work under a contract you view as bad, you perform at less than your best, creating problems for both you and patients. A contract is seldom a "one-shot" collaboration. It will usually be something that you will have to live with, either in its present or renegotiated form, for a long time. In such a situation, you had better be pleased with the results of your negotiations, as should the other signer. (Back to the spirit of win/win.)

The best advice one can give in writing a contract is: Don't be in a hurry to sign. Time taken to check that everything in the contract is clear, free of misleading words or phrases and is fair to both parties will be well spent. Usually the person who writes an agreement derives an advantage. By putting everything that the writer wants in a first draft of the terms that were negotiated, he is in a position of being able to trade for word changes or insist upon his words when they conform to something that was agreed upon earlier. (If you find yourself in this situation, remember that you should get concessions in return for any that you give.) Remember, also, that emotions rather than facts and the feeling that both parties have created something that is useful to both often enter into concluding any agreement. Avoid nitpicking if you did not write the draft agreement; concentrate on the items that are important to you.

There are certain minimum objectives that should be covered in any contract:

- Identify the parties—names, addresses, titles if applicable—and their purpose or intent for entering into the contract;
- Insure that the contract is self-contained; exclude all items that are not written into the agreement;
- List all representations and conditions of work and/or cooperation for the contract to be acceptable to both parties (including adequacy of professional liability coverages, reserves and excess coverages to protect both parties for *negligence* as against *intentional* allegations);
- Delineate the duties and responsibilities of the parties as contractors, payments and payment schedules if any, or fee schedules, cancellation provisions, penalties for non-compliance, and neutral adjudication of differences over contract compliance (including termination);
- Spell out Act-of-God situations for those unusual conditions or unfor-

seeable situations that may prevent compliance under the contract (work stoppages, blizzards or floods, etc.). Be wary of "hold harmless" clauses that slide liability away from the opponent and to you.

- Keep the language as close to "plain English" as possible, avoiding archaic, wordy and potentially misleading phrases.
- Make the effort and offer to write the offers, agreements and other pertinent parts of the contract in layman's language, using as your base the interim written agreements arrived at during the negotiation. Rewrite any boilerplate clauses, if there is any chance of misunderstanding, to be sure that they say *exactly* what you want them to say.
- Put your draft aside for a few days when everything has been completed to your satisfaction, so that when you next read it you can do so with a fresh look. If time is a factor, at least "sleep on it" until the next day. After rereading your draft, go over it once more—looking at the contract from the point of view of your opponent. Ask yourself:
  - Have you put in anything that he might find objectionable?
  - Have all his wants (that were agreed to during negotiations) been included?
  - If you have changed some words or included something to which he might object, is there some other point that could serve as a trade-off?

Contracts being newly written or renegotiated should be approached with the idea of establishing a sound working relationship. Where a contract includes clinical, administrative and other duties it should recognize these diverse objectives by dealing with them separately. For example, a section should describe the specialist/physician as a member of the medical staff, with accountability for his medical work within the organization to the chief of staff and/or the executive committee. Remuneration, either as to amount or method of payment, for either specific or general medical services would be included in this section. Another section should cover the physician's administrative duties and responsibilities, for which he would report to the chief administrator of the organization. Depending upon the amount of time required for the fulfillment of these duties that would detract from the time available for clinical practice and the consequent measurable loss of income, compensation should be included. Finally, there is a certain amount of time traditionally allotted to organization duties on a "volunteer" basis which may or may not be covered in the medical staff bylaws. If the amount of time required by such duties can also result in a measurable amount of monetary loss, salary should be negotiated. Looking at all the preceding from a broad perspective, if the time required for satisfactory completion of the various non-medical responsibilities is full or almost full-time, provision should be made to allow for at least limited practice of the physician's specialty. Be sure to get this in the contract, even if it puts a top limit to earnings, for several reasons. First, it is necessary to keep up-to-date with a specialty, and knowledgeable with what goes on with the practicing professionals. Next, as a full or almost full-time member of the management team, a physician becomes one of "them", no longer viewed by peers as someone with a practice but instead as someone to be kept at arm's length when matters of medical or administrative concern are to be discussed. As long as the limited practice remains limited and does not cut into the regular practices of the practicing physicians, the peer-bond should not be completely lost.

Financial Arrangements

Most contracts concerned with medical practice will evolve among parties where capital investment is or is not required of the physician. The majority of these will relate to hospital-based physicians where no capital investment is at stake. The main concerns of physician signers with these contracts will be with their professional responsibilities and personal financial arrangements. Where capital or investment is part of the contractual arrangement, either by lease, payment of a fixed fee for the exclusive privilege of operating a service, or as an independent apart from the signing organization's establishment, the physicians involved will not only be concerned with professional responsibilities but with fiscal administration as well.

Money is always an important subject in contract negotiations. The subject has become increasingly important because of the increasing subjectivity of third party payors and the complaints to those third parties by the people who pay the bills—employers, government agencies, patients—for cost-effective medical, hospital, and healthcare. Traditionally, financial arrangements in contracts center around a single sum and how it will be paid: annually, monthly, weekly, etc. Even for those physicians negotiating a salary for an employee situation, serious consideration should be given to separating the types of functions being performed and allocating parts of the total monies to those functions. The reason for this kind of thinking is that for a truly cost-effective medical payment system, incentives should be available. Philosophically and practically, people will be prepared to perform at a "satisfactory" level for a set sum. They will even manage to perform at a less-than-satisfactory level, complaining of inadequacies of earnings, administration, and opportunities for personal fulfillment as the reasons for lackadaisical results where there is no opportunity for financial aggrandizement for thoughtful and superior performance. If the job to be done can be divided into measurable functions, bargain for them, with increased remuneration to be received for performance beyond specific negotiated "satisfactory" goals. For cost-effectiveness to be realistic, functions should be reduced to measurable units—office visits or patient contacts per day or other period according to complexity of treatment; ratio of time spent between medical and required non-medical functions such as teaching, inspections, public service, etc.; papers, publications, committee works, supervision, etc.; charges authorized against the organization (lab work, x-rays, prescriptions, etc.); are some of the goals requiring mutual agreement.

For the hospital-based physicians, in light of the various state and other governmental controls that are being established or projected, a two-level system of remuneration is most important. The insurors are most concerned with the increasing availability and use of mechanical devices that perform duties originally done by the physicians themselves, such as SMA 14s, which are run at the cost of a few seconds of computer time, as opposed to the fourteen different time-consuming tests that were performed by pathologists or their technicians. (Of course, here is an area where cost-containment can become a plus for a negotiator: why run fourteen tests when all the attending physician requires is one or two of the total result? And, why run those fourteen tests several times a day or within a short period of time if the patient's condition only requires an overview of a single condition/situation?) If the supervision and quality control of the mechanical aspects of specialty performance can be separated from the hands-on aspects that require knowledge and judgment, it should be done. The responsibility for supervision and quality control, as well as any other overview and control aspects of the position being negotiated, can be assigned a specific sum, subject, of course, to an adequate incentive arrangement. This portion of a physician's function and remuneration should cover all items that, for example, are lumped by Medicare and Medicaid—and followed by the private insurors—into "A" payments to the hospital, which try to include all clinical (technician or machine performed services) work, autopsies, etc. But, while some of these medical functions are treated lightly by the third parties, the physician concerned should place values on his own involvement. That is, pathologists whose work on autopsies is valued as an "A" payment to a hospital should negotiate for an autopsy fee, preferably based on difficulty. Where work is seemingly being paid for by third parties as "scut work" it should be carefully reviewed, if only for the potential time and difficulty involved that would be unavailable for the more important phases of responsibility to a contract and organization.

Despite the prestige and/or ego-satisfaction that come from being known as an "independent contractor," one should look hard at all proposals offered by any organization (hospitals, HMOs, etc.) that invoke that status for an organization-based physician. The way that most contracts are written, the organizations have all the prerogatives of employers and the physician-contractors all the duties and responsibilities of employees, with a series of gross exceptions. While the organizations are able to utilize those physicians as employees, they do not have any responsibility for so-called "fringe" benefits that the employees enjoy. The legal requirements of FICA, unemployment compensation, workers' compensation (including malpractice coverage), pensions, paid vacations and continuing education requirements, dues paid to professional organizations, group life, health and medical insurances, fair compensation on a regular basis, due process, and so on are cavalierly ignored. Perhaps the greatest piece of wool that the organizations are pulling over the physicians' eyes is their callous disregard of due process. Many contracts that I have seen even go so far as to specify that an independent contractor, although required to be an active member of the medical staff, foregoes his rights to the due process that is his under the medical staff bylaws. As a minimum, an independent contractor should have access to the due process available to all the others. Preferably, it should have a combination of "just cause" termination and due process that has, as its final decision-making step, arbitration by a true neutral.

Having made the decision to remain independent, the method of payment becomes important, along with the duties and responsibilities of the job. Flexibility in financial arrangements is desirable. Diversity in size, demographics, and organization make it difficult to suggest one or two "best" types of financial arrangement. Innovation of methods that encourage quality medical care should be fitted both to the physician, the practice, and the demographics of the institution. For those specialties where procedures can be easily delineated and are not too numerous, separate direct billing may be the answer. The institution will want to have some say in the fee structure. The administration will cite numerous surveys that will be constructed to show how much higher the present physicians' fees are than their averages. Any such presentations should be placed alongside your own surveys of current practices. Determine when and under what conditions the surveys were made. You will find that, in many cases, the figures that are presented come from surveys made a number of years before. For example, Dean Grant,[2] in his pitch for complete hospital control of fees and the salarying of hospital-based physicians, quotes AHA and other surveys that were at least seven years old. This is a favorite government tactic, using the publication date (if it is even mentioned) instead of the time—usually three or four years prior—that the data were actually accumulated.

The need to have some form of control over the fees charged by physicians who are contracted with and, in consideration of exclusivity within the organization, form the basis for these arguments. Under pressures from third-party payors, the hospitals have to show that they are doing "something." And the courts, reflecting the public attitude of both open and hidden resentment of apparently fabulous physician earnings, support that thinking. If an organization's efforts of cost control are publicly directed at holding down the physicians' fees and total earnings, it is hoped that those vocal third parties will be less inclined to look closely at how the healthcare institution is doing its pricing. The question that should be answered during negotiations should *not* be what an administrator *thinks* a physician should earn in total but what are *reasonable* fees for the different procedures that are performed and guarantee quality patient care. The negotiators should also distinguish between routine procedures and those procedures where medical training and judgment are the basis for advice and counsel in patient care. The differences between supervision of routine procedures and performance of medical judgment must be understood and taken account of. The former can be looked upon as a consultant retainer, while the earnings from reasonable fees would be performance-derived, and not subject to an administrative conception of what might constitute "fair" income.

Some type of secretarial-accountant service is required to record the procedures to be billed, the procedure for getting the bills to the patient, and the followup for collection. For a fee, the institution usually will be willing to do this. This, of course, delivers some control to the administration, and *requires* some type of double-check on the billing and collection,

---

[2]*How to Negotiate Physician Contracts,* Dean Grant. Second edition, 1983. Teach'em, Inc., Chicago, IL.

thus someone to properly notify the billing service and maintain records upon which to base the checking procedure. Trust and mutual respect are excellent bases for a working arrangement, but the availability of records, dates of payment, credit losses, and periodic accountings, should be in writing.

This advice may sound redundant and perhaps a bit suspicious, but I cannot overemphasize to people who are used to making quick, educated decisions the need for going slowly and carefully. Contracts are made to be lived with for an extended period, and if they contain clauses that can be turned to one of the signer's advantages and the other's disadvantage the adversary relationship that results will affect patient care. So, move slowly, and take time to read and reread your contract before you sign.

Here are some administration proposed clauses that should be avoided whenever possible, or at least so circumscribed that notice and due process are assured:

- Limitations of the administration's liability in the event of accidents not the specific result of the physician's actions;
- Clauses that waive the physician's right to proper and legal notice;
- Restrictions on temporary replacement that could prevent vacations, continuing education, illness, etc.;
- Clauses that place the burden of maintenance or repair of the other contractor's facilities (unless part of a leasing arrangement) or the discipline of his employees assigned to your service on the physician;
- Clauses that allow the other contractor to dictate how you will practice (where not allowed by medical staff bylaws or other professional arrangements) or control your office administration;
- Agreements that waive your right to defend yourself against uncommon proceedings such as joint malpractice allegations;
- Clauses that permit the other contractor to change anything governed by the contract language without consultation and mutual agreement.

Other pitfalls that should be watched for, because failure to avoid them will mean that your contract becomes an unhappy straight-jacket:

- Fuzzy language (covered earlier);

- "At will" termination, perhaps not in your agreement, but in the other contractor's bylaws to which you are subject;
- "Cause" termination not covered by a few more definite explanative words of cause;
- Lack of specifics as to effective dates, continuity while negotiating, automatic renewal if certain procedures are not followed;
- Contract limitations to your rights because of other corporate documents or practices left unspecified in your contract;
- Failure of the governing body to approve the contract in writing;
- Reliance upon oral promises or informal documents offered in wording that was either vague or elusive;
- Contract continuity when, through purchase or merger the party with whom you have contracted is eliminated, opening what may be a contract with considerable time to run to complete cutoff and possibly no renegotiation.

Finally, a *caveat* about the hazards of telephone negotiations, particularly where a contract is the issue. Arm's length can be harmful to your future because assumptions of understandings will usually turn out to be something different for both parties. Verbal agreements may be binding for periods of up to one year. However, should one of you have to take such an agreement to court, facts as well as the circumstances surrounding the making of the contract will turn out to be different than what you thought you had. If you are placed in the position of having to verbalize an agreement out of sight of your contractor, sit down immediately (not tomorrow or a week from the end of the conversation) and write to the person at the other end of the telephone line everything that you agreed to, the way that you understand those agreements. At the end of the letter close with something like: "If you agree that the above is what we agreed to over the telephone, please sign the enclosed copies and return one copy to me." Send two copies of your understandings to the other party via certified mail, return receipt requested. If he does not write or call back with objections, you can, under most circumstances, conclude that what you wrote will hold up. If he does have objections and verbalizes them, and, after discussion, apparently agrees, follow the same procedure of writing and mailing. Get something in writing! *Reliance on verbal promises, particularly when the negotiator has limited authority to commit his organiza-*

tion, leaves you stuck in the quicksand of legalismus. Your greatest leverage comes at the time just before concluding an agreement. That's when flexible understandings can best be tied down, when opalescent promises are translated into an enforceable contract.

Use a lawyer as you work out the details, but not as your negotiator. Let him review the written words, but don't let him overlegalize the language of the contract. *Do not* let yourself be conned into using the administration or organization's lawyers. (No one can be faithful to opposing parties simultaneously, or avoid "conflict of interest" when he is *loaned* out, no matter how vociferously he protests.) And examine a lawyer's expertise before hiring him. For an employment contract, a labor-oriented attorney may be best for you. Certainly you will seldom get good negotiating advice from a probate or tax-type lawyer. And if the person has experience with medical legalese, so much the better.

14

BACK TO BASICS: A SUMMARY OF TECHNIQUES

Everything has been thought of before,
but the problem is to think of it again.
Johann W. von Goethe.

When presenting new material and ideas, it often is wise to recap the major issues. This list offers a quick review.

Fundamental Negotiating Principles:

- *Understanding the fundamental objectives of and for negotiations, both yours and your opponent.*
  -- Opponents negotiate upon assumptions of power potentials of the other side. Maximize that power potential without braggadocio.
- *Strategies during prenegotiation.*
  -- Identify and seek to deal with principals. When possible, identify opponent's weakest member—those most likely to help you reach your goals. (The successful negotiator reaches agreement more quickly, not because he is prone to accept opponents' proposals easily but because he understands opponents' needs.)
  -- Time negotiations to obtain maximum benefits, particularly when your relative power position is at its strongest. (The self-assured

negotiator exhibits informal behavior and casual acceptance of the negotiation process.)

-- Analyze potential goals that you and your opponent might want to reach independently, might be willing to settle for, might have to get.

-- Develop a laundry list of areas requiring research, based upon goals analysis. (Lack of information can be embarrassing, and can be used by opponents to put you on the defensive.)

-- Research data from previous negotiations, where possible.

-- Research strategies and tactics usually used by opponent, types of data used and their credibility, and subject matter areas opponent is most likely to depend upon.

-- Be sure about specifics of laws, regulations, operating rules that may be applicable to goals of both sides, duplicate pertinent elements to have ready in case of divergent opinions.

-- Assure that data researched is pertinent to positions to be taken.

• *Reflections on personal negotiations or use of an agent, team as an audience and assistants.*

-- As your own negotiator, you can be pressured into immediate response, but opportunity to take immediate advantage to tie down better results also exists.

-- Negotiating through an agent serves to shield principals, where principals may be less than capable negotiators. Agents should not be given final authority for decisions, but can feel out opponents for weak spots and arguments. Agents tend to make smaller concessions and larger demands than principal because of the accountability responsibility. Specific parameters, rather than open-ended instructions keep principals in control of negotiations.

-- Using a team as both audience and assistant negotiators permits increased technical expertise, offers opportunity for more observers, and creates feedback with pooled judgments. It also increases the chances of leaks. Internal disagreement and team orientation can be time-consuming and potentially disruptive. Properly used, the team can spread stress in cases of extended negotiations. Where a large group is concerned, a well-knit team can make results more credible when voting for approval of negotiating results.

- *Negotiating strategy and opening tactics.*

  -- Generally, negotiations are of two kinds: your opponent needs you or your services, or, you are in the position of convincing an opponent that he needs you or your services. High expectations will usually pay off in one's favor and require fewer large concessions. If negotiating as a seeker, your opponent must be teased and interested with potentials and benefits before getting into specifics. You may "low-ball" to get opponent thinking in your direction then begin to withdraw and restructure proposal. You may discover some external reason (illegality, other person or party) to withdraw an earlier "maybe" proposal. You may threaten to go over an opponent's head or to make his action public. You may try to impose a deadline to stop stalling.

  -- You may attempt pressure by developing alliances with peers in other specialties who will be negotiating with the same opponent (complicate issues); prepare a *fait accompli* situation for opponent (i.e., if opponent mails a prepared contract, don't negotiate unwanted clauses, cross out bad language, initial crossouts, sign contract and return—may result in opponent signing to avoid negotiation for worse terms).

- *Researching an opponent.*

  -- It's important to know as much as possible about your opponent's operating needs, financial and psychological requirements, how opponent acts under pressure, where potential pressures may be, past negotiation practices. Study minutes of board, annual reports, press releases and advertising, litigation status. Interview peers and others who have negotiated with opponent. Brainstorm and role play using this information.

  -- Double check own data, assumptions, possible reactions to own strategy and tactics (role play).

- *Locale for negotiations.*

  -- Ask yourself where you'll feel most comfortable and relaxed.

  -- Site should not serve to increase tensions (informal), conflict (relaxed), or competitiveness (friendly), but should serve to broaden atmosphere for cooperation and problem-solving (comfortable).

-- Have room to move about, comfortable chairs, air-conditioning (in season), coffee or cold drinks, adjoining room for caucuses.

-- Home, opponent's office, or neutral location? Are you comfortable or uncomfortable in less-than-familiar territory? Host negotiator tends to be more aggressive in own surroundings.

• *Communicating.*

-- Negotitations usually are carried on at three levels: reason and logic, emotions, and subconscious. Communication of negotiator's positions is best when uncomplicated, enthusiastic, fair, truthful, credible, and personal. Communication while negotiating should strive to:

-- Capture and hold opponent's attention;

-- Get opponent interested in topic; presenting it as "our" problem;

-- Develop trust and credibility;

-- Treat opponent as an individual interested in outcome of negotiations;

-- Hold and increase opponent's interest in pursuing negotiations to satisfactory conclusion;

-- Assist opponent's memory retention; and,

-- Stimulate opponent's decision to settle by demonstrating that deal you desire is better than alternative courses of action.

• *Presenting and reinforcing your negotiating positions:*

-- Communicate major points in uncomplicated language, avoiding words that may be heard as equivocal, be as specific as possible;

-- Position should be put as, first, desirable or useful to opponent's situation, then, using examples, stress similarities of positions with pros and cons for both sides;

-- With enthusiasm, present facts and logical assumptions to exploit opponent's motivation and hidden agenda;

-- Satisfy both organizational and personal needs of opponent with knowledge and understanding through cooperative information exchange and problem-solving. Particularly be concerned with his emotional needs for safety, security and self esteem depending upon whether negotiations are going well or poorly for you;

- *Tactics useful in achieving acceptance:*

-- Cooperation in problem solving;

-- Using the "back door"—creating a desire to take a certain action by telling him that you cannot or will not do something ("If I have to do all the things that you are asking, at the limited retainer that you have offered, I won't have time for _____ _____ _____.")

-- Black hat/white hat—tough agent, moderate principal.

-- "Hard to get"—force your opponent to put a value on something that is kept out of reach. If you think that opponent may come up with derogatory statements about you, get them out on the table before he does. By arguing opponent's position he is made to appear stronger than he thinks; you then put out a small concession because of opponent's apparently strong position which may save you making bigger concessions. (Also called "straw man");

-- "Play acting"/"great anticipations"—using credibility, making concessions on contingencies that will probably never take place—presenting a proposal in expectant terms knowing all the time that you will concede only a minimum;

-- "Catch 22"—playing dumb can sometimes be smart. By admitting ignorance of certain issues or phases of issues, opponent appears to sway you with his logic or facts to concede issues that you were always ready to give (also known as "country boy" ploy);

-- "Weakest/strongest"—picking the person with actual authority, directing arguments and rebuttals at this individual, whether spokesperson or not, confer recognition and apparent power to this person when using common sense discussions, giving him opportunity to put aside complex arguments of either side. Directing arguments at person most likely to be disruptive or negative in caucuses;

-- Use of non-verbal signals—listening attitude (when opponent is talking don't interrupt, look interested even when bored stiff. Periodically question to show interest, repeat, return to your position and present alternatives); dead silence after opponent finishes strong position statement puts emotional pressure on speaker to explain further; team changes seating following caucus, team members or chief negotiator gets up and walks about room while opponent is talking to distract speaker.

- *Countering opponent strategies and tactics:*

  -- begin by complimenting, remain calm and deliberate when presenting own views, get mad or abusive only if acting a part, be ready to utilize face-saving gestures (develop a credible excuse for opponent's wrong conclusions or logic—"If I hadn't learned last week that . . . , I'd have felt the same way." or "Perhaps someone put those out-of-date figures together for you."—giving him an "out"—attack the act or language, not the person or, particularly, his ego); humor when everyone is tense;

  -- Design questions to have obvious answers that compliment your positions. Well-formulated queries can diffuse opponents' negativism by exposing irrationalities, and poor logic can put opponent on defensive.

  -- Better to ask questions that require opponent to make a choice than questions that can be dismissed with a yes or no. But, asking a series of questions that keep opponent responding "yes" can be used to build a "yes" attitude when the final question is asked.

  -- If opponent is beginning to bluster, give him a chance to catch his breath, then thank him for so carefully explaining his reasoning, i.e., "I appreciate the time and effort that you have put into explaining your assumptions and positions for this situation. Too few people are so considerate." A mild but sincere approach can cause your opponent to feel foolish and then cooperative.

- *Balancing concessions:*

  -- High, but reasonable, expectations maintained throughout negotiations have a way of producing more favorable results.

  -- Large concessions create suspicion and negative attitudes. A series of small concessions achieves better results.

-- Quick and easy granting of concessions can make an opponent wary and will be seen as a sign of weakness. Spilling one's guts can be dangerous; succeeding incremental revelations do a better job of leading opponent to a desired conclusion.

-- For each concession offered, receive one in return.

-- Test your assumptions of the meaning of concessions for their truth and value early on. This is most easily accomplished by requesting clarification of each assumption.

-- Where an opponent's proposal cannot be agreed to because the concession on your part extends beyond your bottom line, do not delay refusal too long; calmly and logically explain the inequity of his proposal and offer alternatives.

-- *Deadlocks (impasses) real or imaginary:*

-- Deadline ultimatums: may be bluffs, but should remain firm and practice apparent withdrawal from table, offering "if you have any second thoughts on your position, call me" as you leave. (If he does hold out, you can offer to resume negotiations, that the recess has gone on long enough—but you should have some small concession ready).

-- Deadline setting is often effective since time pressures tend to reduce expectations, demands and closing ploys. If negotiations have been fairly productive but are beginning to drag, pushing for a deadline while reminding opponent of all the progress—and all the good things he has garnered—that has been made will make him consider his investment of time and effort and the possibility of loss against completion.

-- If you have been conned into too many concessions, and have taken a hard line reversing some of them to create an impasse, you will affect his investment. This can be the time to demand a few concessions on his part, in return for a less difficult attitude on your part.

-- Impasse may develop when you are having a problem getting your opponent to open up with enough information for you to frame proper answers. The same situation can develop if you are inclined to let negotiations lag somewhat because you are concerned with preserving a status quo. Forebearance becomes delay, and pressures him to open up in order not to lose everything that has been accomplished to date.

-- Finally, if it seems all else has failed to carry your point, the time may have come to act irrationally. The apparent loss of self-control and objectivity can show him that you feel threatened by his attitudes, and that unless he can help you get your emotions under control, the negotiations will come to a standstill.

• *Closing the negotiations—the ultimate purpose.*

-- Knowing when and how to conclude is crucial to the success of your negotiations. By carefully watching your opponent as concessions are made and goals are negotiated, you will develop a feel for the right time. That time arrives when it becomes evident that neither of you is going to make any more concessions and you are satisfied with what has been accomplished. At this point, it is best to sum up your agreements as they have been written, watching your opponent closely to see if there is any semblance of disagreement. *Don't make the mistake of overselling.*

-- When it is time to write the final agreement, offer to put it in draft form:

  • The person who puts an agreement together from scratch is usually more careful about the ramifications of language than the person who reviews a prepared document. This is the time to remember and heed the acronym KISS (Keep It Simple Stupid). After writing, put it aside for a day or two if you have the time, then read it as though you just received it. Ask someone to read it for content, not for style, and forget any pride of authorship.

  • You have the opportunity to prepare or verify the agreement in language that is understandable to you. Particularly if they are the points that are most favorable to you, changing a draft can become an issue of pride of authorship.

-- Be clear upon the means of confirmation of the final draft, and upon who the signatories will be.

15

ARBITRATION: ONE POSSIBLE ALTERNATIVE

It isn't that they can't see the solution,
It is that they can't see the problem.
G. K. Chesterton

Many problems confront physicians when the need for due process arises: delay, confusion, discrimination, imprecision, ignorance or evasion of the documentary record, bungling, self-protection at the cost of truth and justice, and inconsistency. Complicated, timed procedures, with hearings that are often arbitrary and guided by the perpetrator of the need for the due process give credence to the truism that "justice deferred is justice denied." Too often the end result of medical staff bylaws due process proceedings appears Pavlovian; automatic parroting of accusations (frequently given to the accused in obfuscatory verbalese and not in writing) at each succeeding step of the process, each blindly supporting the star-chamber findings of earlier peer groups. Most current due process has become so determined to follow correct procedure that the real reason for the process—the search for truth and justice—has failed to be served.

One option will combine the legal need for procedure and the protection of individual and group integrity. That option is arbitration: the hearing and determination of a case in controversy by a neutral person who has been chosen under statutory authority or by the parties according to a prearranged method. Arbitration serves as an active, needed, and rational area for peaceful dispute resolution. Arbitration also offers an alternate avenue to the expensive, time-consuming, and complicated adversarianism of litigation. It has become widely and increasingly acknowledged as an independent and impartial method that meets parties' requirements for a reasonable assurance of privacy and speedy absolute settlement. Arbitration serves the need of opposing parties for resolving valid disputes by permitting them to determine the method by which their opposing views can be settled most efficiently and productively, without the trauma of judicial determination.

Arbitration as a step in the due process procedure can reduce and alleviate the hard realities of conflict that litigation creates. By having hearings, usually informally, each side is given opportunities to present its interpretation of the issues, with the arbitrator assuming the role of judge. In an arbitration each issue stands on its own merits, without the straitjacket of centuries of precedent, evidence rules, and court formalities. Legal niceties and maneuverings can be put aside, leaving the arbitrator room within which to judge the parties' credibility, causes, merits, and possible solutions for the problems presented to him. With arbitration, parties agree that by taking their apparently irresolvable or emotional dispute to a mutually agreeable neutral, they will accept his decision as final and binding. The interesting thing about "final and binding" is that an arbitrator's decision is just that—there are no litigious appeals available except for very limited reasons. Arbitrator awards may be vacated by a court only: if the award was procured by corruption, fraud or undue means[1]; if it can be proven that the arbitrator was partial or corrupt[2]; if the arbitrator refused to hear pertinent or material evidence[3]; was guilty of misbehavior that prejudiced the rights of parties[4]; refused to postpone the hearing upon showing of sufficient cause[5]; exceeded the powers authorized by the parties[6]; or imperfectly executed his powers[7]. Arbitrator awards may be modified or corrected by a court: where miscalculation of figures or a mistake in the description of a person, thing, or property[8]; where the arbitrator made an award not submitted to the arbitration[9]; or, where the award is imperfect in form[10].

---

[1] 9 USC 10(a); UAA ¶12(a)(1)
[2] 9 USC 10(b); UAA ¶12(a)(2)
[3] 9 USC 10(c); UAA ¶12(a)(4)
[4] 9 USC 10(c); UAA ¶12(a)(4)
[5] 9 USC 10(c); UAA ¶12(a)(4)
[6] 9 USC 10(d); UAA ¶12(a)(4)
[7] 9 USC 10(d); UAA ¶12(a)(3)
[8] 9 USC 11(a); UAA ¶13(a)(1)
[9] 9 USC 11(b); UAA ¶13(a)(2)
[10] 9 USC 11(c); UAA ¶13(a)(3)

Because arbitration serves all disputants quickly, fairly, and inexpensively, some advocates of legalistic stratagems try to disparage and promote distrust of the procedure. Chief among their arguments against arbitration is that the parties will be forced to accept the judgment of an uninformed stranger who has no responsibility for meeting the ongoing relationships of the disputants for the parties' accountable and judgmental interests. If we accept that argument, how much more informed and responsible will a decision be when it comes from a judge or jury after many months and many dollars of courtroom intrigue? The practical reality of arbitration is that although the neutral chosen may come uninformed about medical or healthcare matters, he will not remain uninformed for very long if the opposing parties properly and fully present their facts, positions, and feelings for which all will have been offered ample opportunity.

The only areas that would require an arbitrator with special knowledge would be those concerned with medical competence. Where such knowledge is required, the parties should utilize the services and abilities of a physician accredited in the same specialty as the physician whose competency is being questioned. However, it is the position of the author that any specialist who is requested to arbitrate should not be a member of any medical staff or local society where there may be the possibility of social interaction. An arbitrator-specialist can reasonably be a neutral and more objective one if he comes from an area not less than two or three hundred miles away from the center of the dispute. This procedure can be assisted by either the specialty societies or the American Arbitration Association. Under those conditions, the arbitrator will assume his responsibilities as would a judge.

With a mutually agreed-to arbitration clause in contracts and/or other agreements to serve as the due process protection for the parties, the signatories agree and understand from the outset of their relationship that any disputes or disagreements that may develop during the term of the agreement will be settled quickly, equitably, and in a much less-complicated manner than they would be if forced to litigation. This is, truly, *the* intelligent and professional means for conflict resolution. And, it works.

Here's how. Begin with the basis for due process—the arbitration agreement:

> Any controversy or claim arising out of or relating to this agreement, or the breach thereof, shall be settled by arbitration in accordance with the (Commercial) Arbitration Rules of the American Arbitration Association, (or according to whatever basis for rules the parties may agree to) and judgment upon the award rendered

> by the Arbitrator(s) may be entered in any court having jurisdiction thereof; provided, that should the controversy or claim be a matter of medical competency or judgment, the Arbitrator(s) chosen shall be peer in the medical specialty of the accused, and shall reside and practice not less than two hundred fifty (250) miles distant from the area where the medical controversy or claim is alleged to have occurred.

Another slightly different form of arbitration agreement could be:

> "Any dispute, claim, or complaint arising out of, or relating to the interpretation or the application of this agreement shall be submitted to arbitration under the appropriate Rules of the American Arbitration Association. The parties further agree to accept the arbitrator's award as final and binding upon them. Where medical competency or judgment is the issue at dispute, claim or complaint, the arbitrator chosen shall be peer in the medical specialty of the accused, and shall reside and practice not less than two hundred fifty (250) miles distant from the area where the medical dispute, claim or complaint is alleged to have occurred."

What will be described here is typical of arbitration procedure. Variations will occur, of course, from arbitrator to arbitrator, from tight control of witnesses and representatives to a more relaxed hearing atmosphere. After the arbitrator has been chosen, he will contact the parties to establish the date(s) for the hearing, the location for the hearing, the numbers of witnesses and others who may be involved in the hearing, and make arrangements for the forwarding of any written material that will be common to both parties such as contracts, side agreements, bylaws, etc. The parties may specify that the arbitrator follow a specific procedure, either because one has been written into the agreement or because they have recently agreed upon one. Or, as is more customary, they leave the conduct of the hearing to the arbitrator. Most often, the on-the-spot procedure is established by the arbitrator on the basis of the apparent difficulties of the issues, the number of witnesses, and the hearing room facilities. While some arbitrators conduct hearings that approach the formalities and strictures of a court trial, most arbitrators try to keep hearings as relaxed and informal as an orderly presentation of the parties' evidence and posturings will allow. However, no matter how formally or how relaxed an arbitrator conducts his hearing, he must establish minimum requirements if the award is to be irreversible. As noted earlier, the parties must be given full opportunity to state their cases, have all their witnesses heard, present their evidence and proofs without being cut short, cross-examine the opponent's witnesses and evidence, etc. Should there be a third party with an interest in the controversy, dispute, claim, or complaint at issue, they are entitled to the same considerations, notices and opportunities to participate as are the primary disputants. Everyone with an interest in the outcome of the arbitration must be given the opportunity, within reasonable limits, to present their evidence, and must be offered the time to cross-examine opposing witnesses and evidence.

Formal rules of evidence and similar legalisms are not particularly relevant to the conduct of an arbitration, but may be given consideration by an arbitrator as guides. The burden of proof, in any case, will rest with the party instituting the arbitration. For the arbitrator, perhaps the most important factor in reaching his decision is the credibility of witnesses and the evidence. The impressions that are made by the various witnesses and documentation reinforce his basis for determining the truth or accuracy of the conflicting presentations, as will the conduct of witnesses while testifying and being cross-examined, and the general conduct and attitudes of the parties before, during, and after the hearings. The arbitrator will also consider whether witnesses are speaking with first-hand knowledge, hearsay, or are just repeating gossip. It is the duty and responsibility of the arbitrator to determine, to the best of his ability, the *truth* in regard to all the verbal and material evidence presented. (In the search for "truth" and credibility the more written or visible proof of one's position that can be brought to bear in a hearing, the better the impression of rightness that will be made upon the arbitrator.)

In the search for truth and justice, the swearing of witnesses may be required by local statutes. If not, swearing ". . . to tell the truth, etc. . ." can be put to the parties for choice. Since perjury is not expected, and physicians may be presumed to be honest in their efforts to receive a practical solution to their dispute, the arbitrator will undoubtedly put the question to the parties for decision. Each party comes before the arbitrator as an equal. The arbitrator is only interested in getting from each side its interpretation of the facts and justifications to enable him to make a decision. If the facts are not made available to him, the arbitrator is put under pressure somehow to persuade the parties to clarify the clouded areas so that he will be able to get what he needs to make a proper judgment. (There may be attempts, for reasons best known to a party, to avoid raising certain questions or elaborating upon specific facts. Such avoidance could cloud some of the issues, requiring the arbitrator to intervene, and, in doing so, possibly tend to improve the opponent's potential. This sort of problem usually surfaces when the arbitrator is presented with complex or multiple issues; thus the parties' advocates should not overcomplicate an already exacerbated situation.)

After everyone has been given opportunity to present everything he feels is pertinent to his position, the parties will be given the option of summing up verbally or, because of complexities of the case or because they believe they can do a better job of summarizing their arguments in writing, they may decide to present briefs to the arbitrator. The decision here is usually left to the parties for decision. (If the parties had agreed at the start of the arbitration that they wanted a written record of the hearing(s) rather than depend upon the arbitrator's notes and memory, additional time—and cost—will be required before the transcript is available to all concerned.)

The arbitrator then has a limited time in which to present his decision, normally thirty days. This time, however, does not occur until after transcript presentation and brief preparation and delivery are completed. The end result of the hearings, the award, provides the arbitrator's decision and the remedy that he issues to settle the dispute. That award will be made within whatever restrictions may be in the parties' agreement or submission, but will not attempt to rewrite or otherwise change the parties' written agreements. The arbitrator's job is to *interpret* those agreements and to devise remedies based upon the presentations of the parties and not to legislate or negotiate for them. Whatever way that decision goes, the parties have bound themselves to accept it as final and binding. Although the theory of arbitration is that each case stands on its own merits and is not subject to precedential restrictions or constructions, arbitration decisions may provide benchmarks for the problem-solving of similar future situations. In many cases decisions form the basis for future negotiations between parties having ongoing relationships.

The arbitration process is constructed so that the parties may present their views to an arbitrator themselves. The use of attorney advocates increases the cost both in dollars and time to the parties. However, if one of the parties brings in an attorney as their advocate, the other is almost forced to do so. The reason is that when an attorney-advocate faces a lay-advocate, they come to the table with different thought processes. Lawyers are trained to operate on the basis of precedents that apply to similar situations; the layperson comes to the table concerned with the urgencies of the actions that precipitated the arbitration and tends to apply them on a more personal basis. An attorney, immersed in interpretation of the law and the courts, may devise excellent answers for legal issues without coming close to the basic problem. The lay-advocate on the other hand, will be reaching for a practical solution to the problem at hand. How well either does in appearing credible to the arbitrator may well depend upon the impression the party makes—whether the arbitrator thinks a party is sincere, or merely using legal histrionics, such as badgering witnesses, conducting extensive fishing excursions, or trying to do their preparation through extensive questioning and cross-examination. One of the major advantages of the arbitration process is that it permits the parties at dispute a high degree of personal involvement, flexibility, and self-regulation. As noted, it is private, understandable, adaptable, quick, comparatively inexpensive, and reasonably fair to the particular requirements of parties in dispute.

Knowing all this about arbitration, where should, or can it be put to use?

To begin with, everybody negotiates, although most people may not recognize it by name. Customers seek a better deal, sellers look for a larger order or profit, employers ask for improved productivity and quality, while employees want improved income and security. Physicians must convince patients that certain practices or procedures are necessary for their health, and so on. Following completion of any of these person-to-person transactions, disagreements may occur. Taking such unsolved disputes to law is the usual method for seeking redress or revenge. Arbitration offers the opportunity for an aggrieved person seeking due process to get quick, inexpensive, and unbiased adjudication.

Medical staff bylaws for due process are an example of the advantages offered by the arbitration process. Practically all current medical staff bylaws are in the elaborate and restrictive format recommended by the Joint Commission on Accreditation of Hospitals (JCAH). In practice, each step of that process only serves to reinforce and pass up the decisions made in the initial action taken to discipline a physician. And, effectively in practice, the system serves to follow the napoleonic legal process where the accused is considered guilty until proven innocent. The growing number of court actions instituted by physicians against hospital and medical staff decisions are, to this writer, an indication that there are flaws in the JCAH recommendations. Medical staff bylaws should be revised and updated to include the option for the parties to take their disputes to arbitration as the next-to-last step for due process. Having such an option would eliminate the star chamber mentality imposed by the present procedures and build more and better equity and fairness into medical staff due process. It would also make the process much less onerous and distasteful to the physicians.

Because final and fiscal responsibility for corporate actions rests with its board of directors, insertion of an arbitrator into the due process structure will neccessitate a slight change—to having the decision semanticized to "recommendation." It is normal procedure for a board to accept the recommendations of its appointed administrator for the majority of operation solutions. And all recommendations are made with the understanding that they may be overruled or modified. It is at this juncture that the insertion of arbitration into due process becomes sensible. Cronyism, discrimination, professional jealousy—and other accusations of bias—will be put aside, and fairness will be installed with an arbitration clause as either the last or next-to-last step of the due process procedure. Where recommendations are in order, the arbitrator becomes a fact-finder for the responsible board of directors. His recommendations to the board would, except for some reason of board policy or another valid reason, effectively have the "final and binding" aspect of normal arbitrations.

Other areas in the medical profession that can be well-served by referral to arbitration include: general contract interpretation and/or contract performance (for medical judgment or competence see above); intrabusiness disputes and disagreements (i.e., independent contractor/hospital, group, etc., divisions and/or payments or accounting, partnership performance and/or finances, outside contractors and consultants); patient-physician disputes or misunderstandings; problems or disagreements with third-party payors, medical representatives and myriad bureaucracies. As part of the negotiation process, a phase of the arbitration process called "interest arbitration" is available. Interest arbitration is an impasse breaker for new or renewing contract negotiations. It is not usually encouraged because its purpose is to determine terms and conditions of the contract that both parties will have to live with for the duration of that agreement. It does, however, offer an alternative, best suited, perhaps, to negotiations between groups (management/labor, hospitals/HMOs, etc.).

Referring problems that parties are unable to settle between themselves to arbitration rather than take the extended, expensive, wearying route through the legal system makes sense for today's medical professional. Arbitration offers a viable alternative for unsettled and apparently insoluble problems and disputes. As the old saw says, "Try it, you'll like it."

16

SETTING GOALS: THE UNAVOIDABLE ACTION

. . . One does not know what one knows, or even what one wishes to know, until one is challenged and must lay down a stake.

Thornton Wilder

Common Goal Setting Errors

By now you have read about the process of negotiations and are acquainted with the perhaps undue emphasis on goal-setting. I hope that the results-centered approach impressed you. Experience has shown that, too often, novice negotiators plunge quickly into a negotiation session without carefully considering the ramifications of their goals. Partially prepared, they make just enough mistakes to spell the overall failure of their efforts. To go in without a complete understanding of one's goals achieves both disappointing results and an unsatisfactory agreement. Because the results of effective preparation and well-defined goals are so desirable for satisfactory outcomes, it is essential to weed out goal-setting problems to improve your chances of improving the process.

Unfortunately, producing effective goals is a long and continuing proposition. The problems of goal-setting, whether for an individual or for a group negotiation, generally include disagreements, lack of commitments, incomplete or false analyses of the situations under consideration, inconsistent or unrealistic goals, unclear goals, a know-it-all attitude, and an inability to approach goal setting without emotional involvement.

Whether the process of goal setting is new to you or has been working reasonably well for you, it is reasonable to believe that some of the following common mistakes in goal setting will be useful in pointing out what you should guard against as a reminder of what should be done in formalizing and routinizing goal setting and as a basis for the examination of both your and your associates' goal setting performance. A negotiator will find this accumulation of goal setting errors particularly useful because, if carefully observed, it requires one to consider what may not be being done while at the same time analyzing both the existing and potential goals. During negotiations, sins of omission can have as serious consequences for failing to achieve goals as the sins of commission.

1. **Goals are set too low.** Either the negotiator has not been challenged, his expectations while under a previous contract have been easily met, he has been "getting away with murder," or he hasn't really studied and thought about the ramifications of the work he will be expected to perform under the new agreement. What he is doing is placing his goals at about his bottom line—and the only way he will go in such a planned negotiation is down.

2. **Goals are set too high.** At the other end of the negotiating scale is the person who sets his goals unrealistically high. If such goals are unachievable, not only will the "wisher" fail to come close, he will probably give up early in the negotiation. Goals should be reasonably attainable, embracing one's truly important objectives.

3. **Common goals are not set before individual goals are established.** Where negotiations are being conducted for a group (medical society, partnership, or corporate group, hospital medical staff, etc.) the organization's goals—whether common or strategic—are not always separable into the personal goals of members, partners, or department heads. Organization goals, however reached, must be known to all parties to those goals so that the formulation of individual goals within the organization will be consistent with the common goals. It goes without saying that the common goals must have majority acceptance and minority acquiescence. Common goals identify the limitations for individual goals and potential political machinations while allowing members to express themselves.

4. **Goals for individuals or units are held accountable for conditions beyond their control.** Similar to setting goals too high, the result of goals set in areas where the persons responsible for meet-

ing the goals are not under the control of the party can only result in defeatism and discouragement.

5. **Responsibility for results is incompatible with organization framework.** Where authority is kept separate from responsibility, goals cannot usually be met because the hands of the person responsible are effectively tied. Also, joint allocations of responsibility, or avoidance because no one is in charge becomes the "out," and little is accomplished. Furthermore, if several parties are given joint responsibility, goals are confused because the limits of each person are not defined and the superior/subordinate relationship remains vague.
6. **Work or responsibility allotments are not coordinated with productivity or results.** Too often the nitty-gritty details of a goal are stressed while the reasons behind those details are overlooked. Results and responsibility should be the prime subjects of a settlement.
7. **Goals are inflexible, but are accepted without demur.** Failure to set goals with acceptable variances prohibits establishing potential exceptions when problems arise, creating loopholes for failing to be responsible for outcomes.
8. **Failure to measure both common, routine objectives and readily measurable duties and results.** Where the routine goals are quantifiable or measurable, all parties concerned have a better understanding of what may be involved in the non-routine performances that are the most important requirements of medical performance. Conversely, setting or seeking difficult or unattainable goals can destroy both interest and effort.
9. **Goals may conflict with laws, regulations, or local rules.**
10. **Unresolved differences between members of same side.** Differences of opinion about expected goals and obtainable results may interfere with a positive and sustained approach to negotiations. Differences must be openly talked through and brought to reasonable agreement if a positive and solid-based backing is there to support the negotiator. Everyone, at least in principle, should be committed to the goals and strategies for the negotiations.
11. **Working or operating conditions prevent goals accomplishment because of internal (opponent) problems.** Organization structure and built-in limitations resulting from out-of-date house rules can

produce "no-win" obstructions to smooth working relationships. In this situation, the opponent is inflexibly autocratic. Negotiating for constructive change ("our mutual problem") can be difficult but rewarding.

12. **Failure to set aside inappropriate or currently unattainable goals.** Pride of authorship, weak leadership, and inadequate investigation can combine to put negotiators in no-win positions. Or, failure to allow negotiators flexibility within limits can destroy the possibility of acceptable alternatives. A group must commit itself to a responsible negotiator who is able to innovate. Reality must be the guide.
13. **Symptoms are confused with basic causes.** Goals set to eliminate unpleasant circumstances are often far from the basic cause of the problems. This usually results from a cursory analysis of a situation that overlooks background and attitudes.
14. **Goals become consecrated.** Negotiations seldom proceed according to plan. Flexibility through prepared fallbacks and alternatives must have a place in negotiating plans or negotiators are put into no-win situations.

Preparation is the answer. When you think you are ready to begin negotiations, put aside for a few days all that has been prepared. Then look at it again. You will be amazed to find that questions will be raised that you hadn't thought of.

17

NEGOTIATING BY PHONE: PITFALLS AND POINTERS

When a diplomat says yes, he means perhaps; when he says perhaps, he means no; when he says no, he is no diplomat.

Anonymous

For physicians who would rather avoid face-to-face negotiations, the telephone offers a welcome alternative. Accustomed to handling portions of their practices by telephone, they readily gravitate to it when faced with a task that may become time-consuming. Because most phone conversations are short and to the point, negotiating by telephone seems to be the easy way out of what they visualize will become a series of less than agreeable confrontations. They may be correct—about the time involved. They are more likely to be incorrect—about the economic advantages over the long haul.

The trouble with telephone negotiations is the ease with which misunderstandings can—and do—develop. Avoid the telephone when negotiating matters that are important to you. Let us look at some of the qualities that distinguish how telephone negotiations can work both against and for you:

- **Potential misunderstanding.** Parties can impress each other only with their voices. One's speech becomes all that is available to convince or dissuade the listener. What is missing is the potential visual feedback needed to react properly to what is being said. One is completely dependent upon aural interpretation. This can lead to missing camouflaged meanings and varied interpretations of what is said. If there is no other way to get to face-to-face negotiations, it is best to remember one of Jack London's aphorisms: "Expression is far easier than invention."

- **Accentuated risk.** Because the time allotted to a telephone conversation tends to be shorter than that which is given to face-to-face meetings, the vocal contest of wills is more conducive to a lose/win than to a win/win result. One must be aware that the dangers of a speedy conclusion will be directly related to how well the person called is prepared. When a call comes out of the blue, listen and question for better understanding. Make no counter proposals or agreements if, as the person called, you are not prepared. Postpone any two-way discussions until you have had a chance to evaluate what has been advanced. Time can work in your favor. This is particularly good advice if the subject under discussion is a new one or if this is a negotiation between parties that have not negotiated before. However, if you are prepared and trust your facts and figures, you may feel able to carefully push for a telephone solution.

- **Telephone power.** Initiators of telephone negotiations gain an immediate advantage. The person called will usually have been called to the phone from a work situation and thus is unprepared for negotiations. We can assume that the caller has prepared for this call—he has his facts, figures, and proposals before him and has anticipated potential objections and alternatives. An unexpected call may be a ploy to remove the deadlock from stalled face-to-face negotiations with a "proposition that you can't resist." Can you consider it a credible tactic? Best to listen and question, if necessary, then tell him that you'll call back.

- **Speed, omission and commission.** Using the telephone will, by its very nature, be faster than face-to-face negotiation. Included in the latter will be travel time, face-to-face warmups, and the cost of being away from one's practice, all items that a quick call obliterates. *However,* the easy recompense for saving time and money can too easily result in making verbal errors of omission and commission. The time available and the need to participate in the mutual exchange and exploration of information as well as the impersonality of only vocal contact serve to restrict the comfortable give-and-take of a face-to-face meeting. And the pressure of time that is imposed by the telephone (too often foisted upon an independent physician by bureaucrats who prefer not to leave their offices and wait for deadlines to seek their agreements) can be both frustrating and harmful.

Earlier, I referred to the process of negotiation as involving and concerning more areas than a contract or strictly business relationship. Family relationships, work inter- and intra-relationships, friendships, getting a group together for a golf or tennis outing, or dinner party all utilize the process to some degree. Many of these work and social interactions will be done through the telephone. Frequently the finalization may be put off for a face-to-face approval. But more often the preliminaries and the groundwork are vocalized by phone. The idea is to make the phone phase work for you as much as you can. This can be accomplished by asking yourself a few questions before grabbing the receiver:

- What are the significant ideas and information that I am about to discuss or propose over the phone? Is there an opportunity for certain essential elements to be misunderstood (Do the words I plan to use mean the same things to both of us?) If misunderstandings can take place, would they be better avoided by phone or face-to-face?
- How well do I know the person being called? How credible am I to him and he to me? Is he likely to be more effective than I am on the phone because he spends much more time using the telephone than I do?
- Would I be better prepared for this vocal sparring if I wrote down my important points—and the words I plan to use?
- How much of my information should I extend in *this* call? Will it be better to proceed slowly so I can doublecheck and get feedback on how well he understands my proposals and concerns? Will I do better by setting a series of intermediate goals over perhaps several telephone calls rather than trying to get everything accomplished in one call?
- What words will I use that best define and limit what I am trying to accomplish? What will be his probable answers, objections, and counterproposals? What words might he use to disguise his intent as the conversation continues?

With answers to these questions in mind here are some thoughts to assist you in handling telephone negotiations:

- **Become the initiator rather than the receiver.** Because telephone negotiations are primarily adversary situations, when you receive a call to negotiate immediately and you are neither mentally or practically prepared, tactfully cut the call short. As soon as you have learned what he wants, tell the caller "I'm with a patient (or in some non-interruptable phase of work). When would it be convenient for me to call you back?" By cutting it short and returning the call, you become the initiator.

- **Set your goals and get ready.** As with any negotiation, know what you want to settle for and get your ammunition ready. Determine, if you can, whether the telephone interchange will solve any expected negative reactions as well as or better than face-to-face meetings.
  - -- Have a written list of your goals, arguments and data ready and at hand when you return the call;
  - -- Mentally role play the coming conversation—possible approaches and counters; arrange for *no* interruptions while on this call (if an emergency comes up, cut the call short and return the call at a time convenient to you both; have all your data handy and paper on which to keep notes (memories are too short and subject to too-favorable embellishments);
  - -- Before hanging up, summarize agreements, make notes and offer to prepare a memorandum of the conversation; and,
  - -- Be prepared, at any point in the conversation when the negotiation become sticky, to cut the talk short and hang up. Then quickly get away from the phone while you get your act together.

- **Listen to, and beyond, the words used (his and yours).** Don't hog the conversation, either from habit or because you are nervous—give the person at the other end of the line opportunities to express himself. Listen for the possible hidden meanings behind his words—how the ideas are phrased and spoken, apparent emphasis or deemphasis of words, interest and enthusiasm. In telephone negotiations, even more than in face-to-face meetings, silence after the other party completes a thought can be a most helpful tactic. Extended pauses can make him ramble on with information that he was planning to withhold or to ask questions that tell you some of the doubts he may have about his own position. When you speak, sound interested, businesslike and natural.

- **Get it on paper.** There are those who adopt as a working rule the avoidance of formal written acknowledgment of agreements (What's the matter. Don't you trust me?—Yes, I do, but with all that's going on in my practice, I don't always remember details, so I'm making sure that I do.") However, unless one really knows and respects the credibility of an opponent, I strongly advise that commitments made in telephone negotiations *immediately* be committed to paper and sent (certified mail with return receipt) to the other party. Too often, verbal understandings become misunderstandings, either inadvertently or by choice. And, when misunderstandings are perpetrated, relationships have a way of becoming touchy. As soon as you complete a telephone negotiation, prepare a memorandum of understanding or agreement: "Per our telephone conversation this date, we agreed that: (1), (2), (3), (etc.). I will begin to put these understandings into effect immediately."

The important thought is that *you* do the work. Because you do it, the advantages are all on your side. These advantages to you include:

-- Initiative is yours. You determine the way that the agreement will be spelled out. It is put down the way you understand it. If there is a misunderstanding in the future, interpretation will most likely be on the basis of what you wrote as well as upon your notes upon which the agreement was based. Make sure that you keep the notes you made during the conversations; staple them to your copy of the memorandum.

-- Self-discipline. From a practical standpoint, knowing that you plan to write the memo upon the conclusion of the negotiations, you should find that you listen more attentively and keep better notes than if you were just a participant.

-- Hold the fort. Although you have taken the initiative, the other party may have some objections or additions to your version of the memorandum. The initiative is still yours because the framework of the agreement has been established. Changes can be made within that framework, in most cases reducing the other party to nitpicking, as long as your writeup sticks to the intent of the negotiated settlements. In any case, we are back to the aspect of the *quid pro quo,* since you don't have to give in easily without getting something in return, which should make him less willing to ask for too much.

-- Appreciation. Finally, by taking the initiative, you are in the position of having done something for him lately. After all, you have

> saved him from having to do what may have taken him away from other work.

Negotiating by telephone can be a frustrating as well as a limiting experience. Of course, the occasion can arise when the telephone is essential, especially in a time-proscribed and last-ditch situation, when a face-to-face meeting is not practical. At such a time your voice, your discretion in the use of words, your initiative in supplying valid alternatives, your steadfastness, and your credibility must all come into play. This is particularly the time to question, to pause, to verify and to conclude with the offer to put everything in writing. Remember to approach any negotiation by telephone cautiously.

18

ROADBLOCKS TO AGREEMENT

A verbal contract isn't worth the paper it's written on.
If you can't give me your word of honor, will you give me your promise?

Samuel Goldwyn

Freedom of contract begins where equality of bargaining power begins.

Oliver Wendell Holmes, Jr.

What in the past has been a relatively internal matter between physicians and hospitals and between physicians in various forms of professional cooperation has, because of the mounting public interest in the costs of health care, become a topic of considerable importance. Financial curiosity about all physician costs will undoubtedly continue, but will center particularly on those physicians under contract to hospitals and organizations and on employed physicians as efforts to "contain" hospital cost increases.

When negotiating any agreement with hospitals or other health care organizations it is necessary to understand that those opponents have certain prerogatives and bargaining backups in law. The courts have taken positions that hospitals can restrict the use of their facilities to particular individuals or groups for legitimate business and professional reasons. These include such reasons as the need to ensure that ongoing administrative functions such as quality control, staff education and medical understanding are the responsibility of physicians; administrative control of department scheduling, development of standard routines and familiarity with equipment and personnel are the province of the hospital. Also, with the emergence of corporate healthcare systems, physicians are faced

- **Term.** Open-ended contracts have a way of becoming handcuffs to both parties. Relationships become inert, with modernization and updating something to be avoided. Better to write agreements that have a limited time-span of three to five years than to have one that only terminates at the whim of either party. Renegotiation is good for any relationship, it clears the air and keeps the parties in tune with current healthcare conditions.

Assuming that the person with whom you negotiate is doing so both in good faith and with authority to conclude a final agreement can sometimes serve you poorly. Reliance upon the word of a negotiator who is subject to a superior or a board of directors can result in no contract. Oral agreements may serve one for periods up to twelve months, but no longer. It is best to get everything in writing that will be approved by the final authority. However, even with a written agreement that is solidly signed and properly approved, it could become a damaging piece of paper to you if:

- Fuzzy wording invites an opponent to make interpretations that are detrimental to you;
- The contract is subject to the terms of other documents—corporate bylaws, government regulations, etc.—which could be used to limit your negotiated rights or privileges;
- A clause in an allied document permits termination at will without cause, or for cause that usually covers such subjective reasons as alleged dishonesty, neglect, incompetence, and insubordination, with no reference to due process;
- You signed the agreement with the old management, which is now being told it had no authority to act, and which the new board failed to approve; or
- You relied upon verbalized promises or upon vague and informal notes that only suggested agreement, and, even then, at some unspecified future date.

What all this underlines is that, when you write or discuss another's writeup after negotiations have come to apparent agreement, put it in layman's language. That language should be checked against the memos and other written notes that accumulated during the negotiations. If some of the clauses refer to standards established and accepted by a specialty or healthcare association, it may be advisable to append the appropriate sections to the contract. Above all, if it is necessary to your peace of mind—and don't be afraid to give that as your reason—rewrite any boilerplate or other clauses so that they say exactly what you want them to say.

When you have done all the checking and renegotiating of the semantics, do what many negotiators do; put the draft aside for a few days, then reread it. If time is short, at least "sleep on it"—you may be surprised at what shows up tomorrow. Then, after rereading the agreement, try it once more—from the point of view of your opponent—because good faith is the basis for an ongoing satisfactory relationship. Should something appear obvious to you but has apparently been overlooked by your opponent, point it out to him for correction. After all, a contract that is a good deal for you should also be a good deal for the other party. If it doesn't work for you both, all that the two of you are settling is the framework for future problems.

For convenience, here is a checklist of the minimum items that should be covered in a contract:

- Identification of the parties and their intent for concluding the agreement;
- Complete agreement (self-contained) with all items not included being specifically excluded, unless certain addenda attached are noted;
- Duties, authorities and responsibilities of both parties to be clearly defined or explained;
- Financial arrangements clearly spelled out, with access to records, timing of disclosures, limitations or coverages of professional liability, and possible penalties for non-compliance;
- All benefits that are included if an employment contract (employer-paid FICA, unemployment insurance and other government required taxes, health, life, and long-term disability insurances, pension/annuity programs, malpractice coverage—preferably under a blanket policy, if available—vacations, sick leaves, continuing education leaves, payment of professional society dues, travel expenses and other expenses when for the organization's benefit, available tax shelters, etc.
- Medical staff privileges, including the right to use its due process;
- Specific due process clause (see section on arbitration);

- Termination of agreement, notices for renegotiation including limited automatic renewal, solidity of agreement with any revisions during term to be only when mutually agreed upon, written and signed by the parties.

19

DEALING WITH DRGs

The only prize cared for by the powerful is power. The prize of the general is not a bigger tent, but command.

Oliver Wendell Holmes, Jr.
(Law and the Court, 1913)

In September 1983, the US government established new regulations[1] for calculating Medicare Part A payments or inpatient services on a prospective payment system (PPS) as these relate to Diagnosis Related Groups, or DRGs, to cover *all* non-physician services (including services supplied by outside suppliers). Included are operating costs for routine services, ancillary services, intensive care unit services, malpractice insurance, medical items, and supplies including, but not limited to, prostheses and pacemakers. Hospitals also will be required to ''unbundle'' those services, which for cost reduction purposes, were shared with other hospitals but now will be billed to each user.

Careful study of DRGs by physicians is necessary for self protection and understanding of how prospective payment rates work and affect the practice of medicine. Section 108 of this legislation, for example, gives the Secretary of the Department of Health and Human Services (HHS) authority to establish regulations that will establish differences between medical services that contribute directly to the patient's diagnosis or treatment for

[1]For a useful discussion of DRGs, physicians should read: *Physician's Guide to DRGs*, Robert Shakno, 1984. Pluribus Press, Inc., Chicago, IL.

"reasonable cost" reimbursement under Medicare Part B, and professional services that benefit a hospitals clients *generally* and contribute only indirectly to a specific patient's diagnosis or treatment. In addition, the Secretary is also directed by Congress to establish reasonable cost equivalents (RCE's) that will set limits—or maximum payments for physician services that benefit the general patient population of an institutional provider. What will begin to take shape will be hospital-kept economic analyses of individual attendings' productivity value to the institution. Under such implied pressures, physicians will have to be careful to assure that their standards for quality care are not compromised or short-circuited by hospital financial administration while treating specific cases.

The physicians should understand that in effect the new legislation puts HCFA, insurance carriers and hospital administrators in the saddle in determining what are and are not physician services. Their decisions could be self serving. When negotiating, you may want to try for arbitration where bureaucratic determinations conflict with services authorized and recognized by the state. Such conflicts will not be easy to win.

On the surface, HCFA's concern is provider cost effectiveness (read cost reduction) through prospective reimbursement. With DRGs, HHS has begun to make redundant the innumerable individual variations required for quality medical care by establishing a system of broad-based case-type payment. With prospective reimbursement, hospitals will be trying to outguess next year's costs on then current bookkeeping. For the institution-based physician, the squeeze is on because from now on he will be competing with *all* the inhouse pressure groups subject to the board of directors. And, under the pressure of DRG restraints, physicians undoubtedly will find that hospitals will begin to insist that particular phases of patient care be serviced in the doctor's office rather than in the hospital where such care would possibly result in financial embarrassment.

If this makes the future look grim for the profession, it shouldn't. Few doctors were in favor of Medicare or Medicaid when those laws were passed, but the potential was quickly seized and put to benefit. What physicians do with the present apparent roadblocks will depend on hospital and patient relationships. Hospital-based physicians will have to develop a radical restructuring of their contractual relationships. Negotiation will become more important; the individuals concerned will have to become more directly involved with the nitty-gritty of their contracts and not depend upon hospital administrators or their attorneys for protection and help. The pattern of past bargaining has been accommodation because costs under "cost-plus" reimbursement were not seen as too important.

The pattern of future bargaining will become more self-oriented because each party will be reluctant to compromise within the opponent's bargaining framework. Complying with HCFA regulations while remaining a viable institution will make hospitals tend to treat their medical constituents more as employees than as partners.

While HCFA currently sees its primary problem of hospital-based physicians as dealing with pathologists, anaesthesiologists and radioligists, the growing number of independent physicians working as part-time independent contractors in specialties that are dependent upon hospital-owned equipment must also be aware of their need to negotiate reasonable working agreements. Perhaps the time has come when some of the free services that have been traditionally performed by members of the medical staff for the benefit of the hospital should be reviewed and updated to the realities of TEFRA. To sit back and take it will only give impetus to the foreseeable increase of adversary attitudes presently exhibited by both government agencies and other third party carriers.

What are some potential areas for negotiation and clarification? Begin with the ever present problem of alleged malpractice. The way Medicare and Medicaid, as well as most insurance programs, have been managed, reasonable costs have been covered with the patient able to get almost everything he asked for—"the best available care." With DRGs as a combination guide and reimbursement limit, much of the "defensive" medicine that has developed to counter ambitious attorneys and contentious patients from going, or threatening, to take their cases to court will undoubtedly become subject to the fiscal determinations of administrators. Should additional tests or procedures be necessary and documentable, but not allowed by the hospital because of the DRG limit, and a malpractice case ensues, shouldn't the hospital become liable, either solely, or at least jointly? This thought, understandably, has yet to become a problem, but it would be useful to bring it to the attention of your hospital and have in your contract some sort of quit-claim that would absolve any allegations of liability where hospital rules limit patient care costs.

Another area of potential misunderstanding will, I believe, become the ethic and fundamental of medical practice: quality care. Without doubt, circumscribed delivery of medical care within the limitations of DRGs to hold down hospital costs will reduce the flexibility and, perhaps, the interest in searching for proper diagnoses and treatment of patients whose problems exceed the average proscribed by the DRGs. As greater emphasis is placed upon DRG payment, physician income will most likely assume the status of employee piece-rate remuneration. If that seems to be the direction an administration is heading, some form of incentive should be built into a contract. Profits or decreased losses attributable to one's specific practices or department operation, number and/or frequency of cases and/or procedures above a specified average of a number of previous years, even implemented suggestions for profitable institutional change are some areas where additional individual income might be generated.

Because medical records probably will become the major basis for Medicare and Medicaid payment, another area of potential adversarial argument may develop over who has the final say about principal case diagnosis for the DRG. Physicians will, as the patients' accountable concern, insist that they and not someone in medical records should determine what goes into the records. It is possible that hospital administrators, in the name of expediency and improved cash flow, may authorize medical record coders to determine or change principal diagnoses that were reported by physicians. Contract language should be included to deny the coder the right to change or determine a final diagnosis without prior consultation *and* approval. What will be required, of course, is that each physician become totally knowledgeable of the DRG terminology associated with his specialty as well as some understanding of peripheral DRGs that impinge upon that specialty. Also required will be greater attention to patient chart upkeep because unlisted diagnoses (left out for whatever reason) can result in downgrading a DRG.

With the pressure of dichotomization upon provider and medical services that ". . . contribute directly to the patient's diagnosis or treatment. . ." there will flourish all kinds of suggestions—both in the literature and on the golf course—on how to upgrade DRGs. Granted, the databases for local DRGs may be less than accurate in terms of up-to-date data. Diagnoses have been classified into 23 major diagnostic categories based on organ systems, and then into 467 distinct groupings that are "medically meaningful." A physician should not use this tactic; consciously playing such a game can only be self-defeating. If administrators and accountants want to take that road to cash flow, let them. Being ordered to do so raises another negotiating issue. What has been done fairly and signed for should be left alone. Any suggestions for systematically coding diagnoses to maximize hospital reimbursement should only be accomplished—if one feels that he must—after getting the order, whether general or specific, in writing or on tape. There will be multiple ongoing investigations, because trust seems to be more and more a thing of the past, and getting caught in such revisions will do no good to anyone's reputation.

For those duties that fall into the ". . . contribute to the benefit of a hospital's patients generally. . ." that have, to now, been part of the total remuneration for hospital-based physicians, compensatory revaluation of the extent of work required should become part of the negotiations strategy. These would include: supervision and quality control management of the recommendations that result from work ". . . frequently and consistently performed by non-professional personnel. . ."; responsibility for the results of such non-professional personnel; training of such personnel; consultations and follow-up of Part A classified results; and any other specific responsibilities that have become part of the physician's departmental work. Under prospective payment systems, responsibility for the maintenance of quality of care is delegated to Peer Review Organizations (PROs), which will review the:

a. validity of diagnostic information offered by the hospital for the purposes of DRG verification;

b. completeness, adequacy and quality of care;

c. appropriateness of admissions and discharges; and

d. appropriateness of care provided to "outlier" cases (unusually long lengths of stay with costs substantially above the DRG rate).

When negotiating for responsibility compensation, a physician must include getting written authority that will permit him fulfillment of the responsibilities that the hospital is requiring. Without authority, responsibility will only become the albatross an administrator will willingly use to clear the hospital of allegations of mal- or mispractice. There is a fine line to be drawn when insisting upon authority. A supervisor carries inclusive authority in relation to immediate subordinate hospital employees. Hiring, firing and disciplinary actions will be available under the specific house rules and personnel policies. However, if one is a contracting physician, such actions may be limited to recommendation for action by the hospital authority. When such recommendations are made, preferably in writing and with sufficient documentation, they should be handled expeditiously by the authority responsible for personnel of the hospital.

Given the crutches of TEFRA, DRGs, and RCEs on which to lean as excuses for disciplinary or oppressive action, hospital attorneys will undoubtedly propose contracts without avenues for due process. Turnover of professionals on staff, whether employees or independent contractors, may well be accelerated by the willingness of non-staff physicians to accept remuneration that will return more to a hospital's coffers. Those ninety- and one hundred and eighty day notices (ostensibly to serve the wills of either party, but really for the hospitals' convenience) can become bear traps without viable due process. Ability to remain on the medical staff—usually automatic removal follows contract severance—should be built into a contract so that the medical staff's bylaws due process remain available, if that route to justice is desired. As a member of the medical staff, provided one's relations with other staff members have been healthy, removal from a contract position may still offer opportunities for consultation and practice. Provided the reasons for severance were financial, a case might be made against exclusion from practice in a hospital granting exclusivity if qualifications can be sustained because of one's previous excellent record. Arbitration, covered earlier, should also become part of a contract.

A new era of hospital-physician relations is beginning. Similarly, a new era of physician-insuror and patient relations is at hand. As very visible—and envied—subjects of political cost control and containment, physicians will have to be much more careful of their contractual relationships than they have in the past.

20

STRATEGIES AND TACTICS: TWO CASE STUDIES

General propositions do not decide concrete cases. The decision will depend on a judgment or intuition more subtle than any articulate premise.

Oliver Wendell Holmes, Jr.
(Lochner vs. New York, 198 U.S.)

A negotiator begins work in much the same way that a novelist does—with a clean sheet of paper and an idea. And, as the writer's ideas develop and take form, the clean sheet becomes covered with words, sentences and paragraphs interspersed with revisions. In similar fashion, negotiations progress: ideas become proposals and counterproposals, with the opponents, hopefully, practicing give and take to a goal of mutual understanding and satisfaction.

The following cases are presented to show that the basic principles in this book can be applied to almost any situation. Obviously, details and circumstances will seldom be the same because both opponents and situations will vary as circumstances change. How negotiations proceed will depend upon opposing objectives and strategies, and the willingness of the parties to hold fast or compromise.

With the situation before you:

- Establish your objectives;
- Set up a strategy or series of steps that will promote movement toward those objectives;
- Negotiate.

Situation 1

You have been in private practice for fifteen years in an average size community and, with twelve peers practice the same specialty (along with ninety-five other physicians) in the town's major hospital.

During rounds this morning, a physician-friend questions you to learn if you had heard the rumor that promoters of a Health Maintenance Organization (HMO) had been negotiating with the hospital for its use by their potential patients. You had not. After rounds, you meet the hospital administrator in the corridor, put the question to him, and learn that the rumor is true. The administrator adds that he believes that HMOs are "the wave of the future," and adds that the hospital will have to associate with the HMO if it is to survive in view of public concern with hospital costs and expected government cost containment regulations. He concluded the conversation with the comment that if the medical staff did not go along with the program worked out between the hospital and the HMO, the HMO might well take away patients by hiring salaried physicians.

After returning to your office, you make several telephone calls, including one to the regional Health Systems Agency (HSA). After a good deal of questioning you learn that the new HMO, when approved, will be funded with seed money of $3 million by the HHS for feasibility studies, low interest rate loans, access to government surplus office, and other equipment. You also learn that the promoters of the HMO are already in negotiations with the management of the automobile parts plant to provide pre-paid health care to its 2000 plus employees.

You contact a number of your colleagues. Most of them tell you that they have already been contacted by the HMO promoters with invitations to join their panel of providers. No one seems too anxious to disclose the financial arrangements. One physician reports that the HMO people offered him an RVS unit value of fifteen for the HMOs' private patients, and a conversion value of ten for Medicaid and Medicare patients. (From another source you learn that, in order to get the seed money and grants, the HMO promoters expect over one-third of the expected patient rolls will come from patients on Medicaid, other federal and local welfare programs, with the expectation of at least another 20 per cent to be Medicare recipients.) Another of your peers admits that he had been offered an RVS unit value of nineteen if he will sign immediately, even though it is generally known that he plans to retire within the coming year. (The average RVS factor being paid by private insurors in the area is twenty—a well-known fact.)

Confused and disturbed, you call your attorney to find out if all this maneuvering is legal. His response: "Well, yes, and again, no. You can always bring an antitrust lawsuit against the hospital, the HMO and its promoters but your chances are at best less than 50/50, and you can look forward to years of expensive litigation."

That night at home you work at your typewriter, writing long letters to the Secretary of the HHS, the President, your Senators and your Congressman. The next morning upon reexamination, and with considerable urging of your spouse, you deposit the letters in your round file.

After rounds the next day, you meet the president of the hospital medical staff and learn that the HMO promoters and their honorary chairman, a physician, have been invited to address the medical staff at its next quarterly meeting—two months hence. Your comment: "That's closing the barn door after the cows have been stolen!"

Objectives

Obviously, no one solution can resolve this situation. However, before establishing your objectives, a few preliminary things should be worked through. First, take note of the incidents described in the situation. It seems obvious that the hospital administrator is *not* being completely above board with the medical staff—physicians are being approached separately with non-uniform proposals. So, if the administrator is trying to divide the staff and accomplish the hospital's alignment with the embryonic HMO, the first task will be to coordinate the doctors to undertake some form of concerted action. (There appears to be two months before the HMO gets to talk to the staff.) Rather than repeat here at length about the process of organization, remember or reread the chapter on organizing. The physician group in this situation will not be organizing to become a union-type assemblage, but it must be prepared to negotiate with the hospital, the HMO, or both—as a cohesive unit. One caveat, here. Get a positive commitment from your colleagues, a financial one.

With the physicians committed to a defense for continuing in private practice, although perhaps in some form of contractual relationship, the group should set some preliminary goals. Preliminary, because you need a lot more information before you can set positive goals. For instance: Who or what organization(s) are behind the HMO?; How do HMOs work in other areas vis-a-vis physicians?; Can we maintain our practices with private patients while servicing HMO subscribers?; What is the record of the HMO movement, have they been successful and/or profitable in communities like ours and how have the private practice physicians in those areas met the challenge? Will cooperating with the HMO and the hospital in their efforts at cost containment affect our medical practices and judgments, will we be subjected to "cookbook" practices? All this, and more when the questions from the group begin to flow.

Obviously no one will be able to answer all the questions to the majority's satisfaction; research is the next step. The staff leaders should spread the work around, create committees, assign projects with definite goals, and set time constraints for results. Then follow up, keeping loosely in touch to be able to either assist or advise. With the answers to your questions at hand, and made available to the group, you are ready to set goals.

What will these be? First, the need to maintain a uniform and concerted front before the hospital and the HMO—all approaches to individual physicians to be listened to without positive response and immediately passed on to the negotiating committee. Next, the need to maintain individual practices regardless of the commitments that may be made with either the hospital or the HMO. Then, uniform contracts; equalized payment practices; due process procedures to encompass both problems that may develop between physicians and the HMO or hospital in the administration of health care, and so-called disciplinary actions resulting from differences in medical practice with HMO directives; set up arrangements to police HMO and hospital conformity with agreement; and any other objectives that may be indigenous to the local staff.

Strategy

Take your time in negotiating, with the proviso that any major agreement has to be approved by the staff as a whole. Have individual members use their contacts with hospital board members for information. Keep the medical staff informed, with two-way communication between staff members and the negotiating committee and a united front (and with any dissension or disagreements—that are bound to develop in a collection of independent-minded physicians—to be kept within the group, unpublicized, for that purpose). Have all proposals of the opponents checked by a qualified (labor or independent) attorney for legality, for what is best for the staff, and for possible alternatives.

Negotiate

When negotiating, don't forget to caucus occasionally to be sure the team is together and to review the other side's approach. Stay calm, and question—particularly when your research can be used to effect. Report to your constituency, taking referenda when necessary to accept or reject potential agreements. Final agreement should be made upon acceptance by the medical staff.

What occurs during the process of negotiating can depend, in large part, upon the suppression of personal fears and ambitions of the members of the medical staff. Comfortable practices, steady income, status and respect may well be viewed as already lost to the power and financial backing of both hospital and HMO. These can be counter-described as arrogance and potential bankruptcy through opponent greed and mismanagement. If the medical colleagues agree to reconcile themselves to changing times and conditions (as did the medical profession with Medicare and Medicaid after fighting a losing battle in Congress and the media), they will be better prepared to work toward an equitable solution to this dilemma.

Predictions are always difficult, especially about the future.

Nils Bohr

Situation 2

You are the senior of seven specialists who have privileges at a prestigious teaching hospital and you have been serving these past few years as the department head for your specialty. Several years ago the board hired the present administrator to update the hospital administration and eliminate recurrent and continuing losses. One of those changes was the hiring of a full-time medical director to oversee the work of the medical staff and to serve as liaison between the board and medical staff to implement the board's policies established for the staff.

The medical director has decided that the hospital administration will be more responsible in running its medical affairs if the department heads are hospital-appointed and paid on a part-time basis, and has asked you to accept the post of clinical director. His description of duties was, at best, sketchy, with his emphasis being placed upon the need for coordination, quality care and patient safety. He did emphasize, also, that the work should not interfere with your regular practice.

You ask what other clinical services will be established and who are being asked to head them. The answers were vague: "We're still in the planning stage.'' You ask for time to think about the proposal and set a date for three weeks from now.

Objectives

Before setting any objectives you will have to decide whether you would seriously consider taking on the responsibilities that will add to work time that is already full. As Samuel Butler once wrote: ''If you would do good, you must begin with minute particulars.'' With the tentative offer of part-time employment to consider, a number of questions should be answered before setting objectives and entering into negotiations. And the questions should establish a base for research. Questions that quickly come to mind could include:

- How will this affect my practice and my relationships with my peers on the medical staff?
- Do I want to become an administrator and, am I qualified either by experience or temperament to handle a job that may require being a watchdog over my peers?
- How much time, and at what hours of the day(s), will I have to be at the job?
- Will the compensation cover lost income because of time away from my practice?
- What will the duties of a part-time department head be—will there be a job description or will there only be vague parameters within which I will be expected to create the job?
- Do other hospitals in the area have similar positions, how do they operate and what do they pay? Are there writeups on those jobs, and who holds them?
- What are the benefits that may accrue to such a part-time position? Will the hospital offer the same employee benefits, or at least pro-rata benefits on the basis of time involved?

The decision to accept or decline the offer need not be made at this time unless you have already decided to refuse. Depending upon the answers that come from your research, your objectives at this stage need only be to get definitive answers and projections from the medical director and the administrator. With a better understanding of what will be expected, your decision to negotiate or not can be made. Then, objectives can be developed.

Assuming that you are going ahead, some of the goals you may want to set should probably include:

- Job definition—who appoints, to whom responsible;
- Primary duties and responsibilities, secondary duties and responsibilities (in writing);
- Authority—discipline (who and under what conditions), appointments, relationships within medical staff and administrative personnel and hospital personnel;
- Accountability—reporting, quality of medical care, changes in privileges, professional performance, discipline, patient safety, programs, etc.
- Time required—minimum and/or maximum;
- Reimbursement—both for time required as above, and excess time, when required;
- Reviews;
- Provision for due process;
- Benefits, parity with other employed professionals (at least on pro-rata basis);
- Maintenance of private practice.

Combining your research and objectives, you are ready to plan your strategy. The major problem will be to separate the promises and/or maybe's from the solid committments that come through negotiations, and to get agreed-upon results in writing (in those areas where the hospital negotiator tries to remain vague or or refuses to commit anything to writing, follow up immediately after the negotiating session with the memorandum to the negotiator with your understanding of those items favorable to you). Plan to push the hospital negotiator to do most of the talking, using questions to put your objectives on the table. Remain calm during negotiation sessions. After all, you're in the driver's seat—they want you.

APPENDIX A
THOUGHTS TO CONSIDER BEFORE, DURING, AND AFTER NEGOTIATING

The chains of habit are too weak to be felt until they are too strong to be broken.

Samuel Johnson

It's impossible to find the exact formula for successful negotiations and win/win outcomes. However, certain fundamental practices can give you a better chance at favorably resolving those issues that have the strongest impact on you and on your patients' care. The list that follows contains items that are important to pay atention to before, during, and after negotiating.

- **Negotiating is neither a stable nor an unchanging process.** It requires planned behavior, realistic conjecture, credible facts and analysis, close attention to words, attitudes and emphasis, logical presumptions of opponents' actions and presentations, as well as presentations maximized for effects.
- **At any stage of a negotiation limited opportunities exist for achieving the best deal possible.**
- **Before entering into a negotiation understand your reasons for doing so.** Examine those reasons to establish bottom lines and potential concessions. With these in hand a negotiator is more likely to be

flexible as negotiations proceed, and concessions and goal stresses are more easily handled.

- **Planning must include comprehension of opponents' psychological and institutional needs as well as their past use of strategies, tactics, and their strengths and weaknesses.**
- **Role playing as a part of preparation can make an actual negotiation a more comfortable exercise.**
- **When negotiating against a team effort, work on the weakest member for concessions or disruptions while maintaining your own team control and discipline.**
- **When negotiating through an agent make your goals, bottom lines and potential concessions absolutely clear and define his limits of authority.** Agents held strictly to accountability generally make fewer concessions and heavier demands than do negotiators who are personally involved.
- **Try to negotiate when you are in your strongest position and your opponent may be at some disadvantage.**
- **Negotiations are best conducted when progress is kept quiet and within the negotiators' framework, and without an audience.** Observers, particularly when they have a vested interest in the outcome of the negotiations, will manage, or at least attempt, to influence their negotiators to avoid concessions and to hold unpalatable positions.
- **Agents can be tougher negotiators.** They can be irritating and adversarial to opponents, because after the negotiations are completed they are no longer part of the working scene, leaving their principals the "nice guys."
- **Trust, workable relationships and credibility result from initiation and maintenance of cooperative and supportive conduct in the early stages of a negotiation.** Conversely, competitive conduct invites reactive competition and an adversary relationship that can drag out negotiations but must eventually be overcome. In short, actions invite reactions.
- **Early on one must become aware of opponents' needs and hidden agenda.** But knowing is not enough; one must show sincere interest in those needs by recognizing them as subjects that have to be discussed

and solutions sought, as part of one's game plan. Problem-solving works to invite opponents to cooperate in searching for mutual advantages and solutions. Win/win is *always* better than win/lose or lose/win and can reduce the time required for negotiations.

- **Negotiating surroundings and conditions should be kept comfortable, relaxed and as tension-free as possible.** Informal discussions before the actual confrontation at the bargaining table may be helpful to define the areas of disagreement and agreement.
- **"Non-negotiable" demands usually develop arbitrary reactions and create intangible side issues that make eventual agreement difficult.**
- **In the early stages of a negotiation work on the least controversial issues to develop a spirit of cooperation.** Financial issues should not be taken up, and certainly not settled, until most, if not all, non-financial issues have been agreed upon (too often, settling financial issues early on will result in bypassing important non-financial problems as "not important" or "we'll take care of that when it becomes an issue"). Early in negotiations is a good time to make small concessions, because it creates an impression of the other negotiator's power and lays the groundwork for getting cooperative (quid pro quo) concessions. Intimations of potential gains can induce him to entertain your point of view, and by inviting his interest you have a better chance of not making him into an active adversary.
- **Negotiations are simultaneously carried on through several levels of communications; reason and logic, emotion and subconscious.** No matter how reasonable and logical you feel that your presentation may be, if it is not understandable and attractive to the listener it may not register as you wish it to. Stress the similarities of goals and intent rather than the differences and make your point at the end of the presentation. This kind of lead-in to your basic goals will then remain in his memory.
- **The opponent's habits must be learned and catered to in order to avoid antagonizing or intimidating him.**
- **Eyes and mouth are a negotiator's most revealing non-verbal communication tools.** Look directly at an opponent when speaking; avoiding direct looks may make him feel that you are insincere or unsure of what you are discussing. Smiling is easier than frowning;

looking directly at him with understanding will promote a much more cooperative attitude even if the subject being discussed is unpleasant. (Occasionally, when faced with a loud and obstreperous opponent, a good tactic is to start smiling, work into chuckles, then laugh out loud. "What's so funny?" "You. You should see the way you look when you act this way.")

- **The apparently obvious issues of an opponent's negotiation effort often obscure his underlying thoughts.** These should be discovered and brought into the open, can sidetrack negotiating progress. An opponent's psychological needs for esteem and survival (particularly with bureaucrats like hospital administrators) may evade the logic of your presentation until and unless his value systems are properly dealt with.
- **Seek solutions by working together.** Problem-solving is most effective when you get your opponent to join with you in seeking solutions and getting away from each party only talking along his own track.
- **Listening can help to satisfy an opponent's ego, showing that you are appreciating and trying to understand his presentations.** If he feels that you are ignoring or casually misunderstanding him he can become openly adversarial. After showing that you recognize the parts of his presentation that do not deflect your goal achievement, suggest your views in a manner and with words that do not belittle or deny either his statements or his goals.
- **When, in doubt about anything that is being said, QUESTION!** If you feel that what you are saying may be subject to misunderstanding or your opponent looks doubtful while you are making a point, EXPLAIN!
- **Third parties, preferably neutral, can help negotiations.** They can serve to clarify differences that are creating impasses into problems that may be solved, can offer face-saving opportunities by suggesting corresponding mutual concessions, and, if nothing else, can keep the parties talking.
- **Because the process of negotiation is particularly sensitive to the intricacies of conversation, each party's actions are extremely contingent upon his perceptions of the other's moves and presentations.** Any aberations in the communication links that can affect the information available about the other side's intents and beliefs and thus distort interpretation of those actions could have major implica-

tions for the eventual solution. Cooperation in problem-solving naturally increases as opportunities for and the use of communications are expanded.

- **A good negotiator demonstrates viability through the following characteristics:** he should not feel the need to be liked; but should be able to command the respect of his opponents and peers and be sensitive to their feelings; he should think and verbalize logically and understandably; he should be able to listen constructively while maintaining creativity and flexibility; he should be able to remain calm and alert during the crush of negotiation and exercise good judgment while making decisions; and he should be able to maintain working relationships, especially in tough situations.
- **As agreement is reached on various issues during negotiations, it is to the advantage of a negotiator to prepare interim write-ups.** When agreement in principle for the total agreement has been reached a final advantage can be had by offering to, and by writing, the draft agreement for final approval of the parties.
- **After an agreement has been finally certified and signed, vigilance is needed to be certain that both parties are observing its terms and intents.** Notes and all supplementary interim agreements should be filed and available for reference should any differences arise during the term of the agreement, and for preparatory research for future negotiations.
- **When negotiating with representatives of bureaucratic organizations, learn and know the rules, procedures, practices, and inconsistencies of the organization.** Because bureaucrats neither want to have waves disturb their equanimity nor the people who create them, a competent negotiator simultaneously introduces elements of personal jeopardy for an opponent while offering the potential of praise for his opponent to his superiors if bureaucratic red tape or internal operating contradictions can be eliminated. By playing to their self-interest while intimating possible embarassments, a negotiator retains control of the direction of meetings to introduce viable alternatives.
- **Finally, strive to remain at least outwardly calm at all times.** Do not take things personally—observe the source and search for the rationale. When you decide that your act requires anger, humor or surprise *act* it. Above all, be comfortable with your presentations, questions and expectations; be flexible and alert, and you will do better than if you aren't.

APPENDIX B
COURSE OF ACTION

Chapter 4

Scenario 1—Suggested Course of Action

Identify the problem and ask yourself how it will affect your corporate and individual earnings and relations with the hospital and patients.

Other methods of payment for the patients or the hospital. Some possibilities:

1. Salary
2. Fee-for-service
3. Lease the department from the hospital
4. Fee-for-service with minimum guarantee from the hospital
5. Fee-for-service with independent contractor payments for ''A'' type services performed for hospital-received payments

Check with national specialty societies, AMA, AHA, and JCAH for similar problems and current solutions. Talk to your peers who are involved in the specialty area. Contact a competent negotiator (labor attorney). Prepare your strategy and alternatives. Negotiate.

Scenario 2—Suggested Course of Action

The medical staff needs time to organize for compliance. Visit the administration and request an extension. Appoint a committee that, with the approval of the incoming chief of staff, will:

1. Study and compare the old and hospital-prepared bylaws;
2. Contact state medical society and the AMA for direction and assistance;
3. Contact JCAH for explanation of their charges. What is the minimum required for compliance? Ask for extension because of the unprofessional approach of the board.
4. Call a compulsory meeting of the attending staff physicians at which you present the situation and the problems.
5. Check with members of other hospital staffs to see what they have done or would do in similar situations.
6. Prepare an alternate set of bylaws with the help of a qualified attorney (not the hospital's attorney).
7. Appoint a negotiating team with the approval of the incoming chief of staff.
8. Prepare for negotiations.

BIBLIOGRAPHY

Alinsky, Saul; *Rules for Radicals;* Random House, New York, NY, 1971.

Bellow, G. & Moulton, B.; *Negotiation, The Lawyering Process;* The Foundation Press, Mineola, NY, 1981.

Berne, E.; *Games People Play;* Grove Press, NY, 1964.

Brown, L. M.; *How To Negotiate A Successful Contract;* Prentice-Hall, Englewood, NJ, 1955.

Cadmus, R. R.; *Hospitals Are Us;* Teach'em, Inc., Chicago, IL, 1979.

Cohen, H.; *You Can Negotiate Anything;* Lyle Stuart Inc., Secaucus, NJ, 1980.

Conflict Resolution In Today's Economic Climate; Proceedings, Ninth Annual Meeting, Society of Professionals in Dispute Resolution, Washington, DC, 1982.

Druckman, D. (ed.); *Negotiations;* Sage Publications, Beverly Hills, CA, 1977.

Dyer, W. W.; *Pulling Your Own Strings;* Thomas Y. Crowell Co., New York, NY, 1978.

Farmer, R. and Associates; *What You Should Know About Contracts;* Arco Publishing Co., Provo, UT, 1969.

Felsenfeld, C.; *Writing Contracts in Plain English;* West Publishing Co., Minneapolis, MN, 1981.

Grant, D. E.; *How To Negotiate Physician Contracts;* Teach'em, Inc., Chicago, IL, 1979.

Gulliver, P. H.; *Disputes and Negotiations;* Academic Press, New York, NY, 1979.

Ilich, J.; *Power Negotiating;* Addison-Wesley Publishing Co., Reading, MA, 1980.

Ilich, J.; *The Art and Skill of Successful Negotiation;* Prentice-Hall, Englewood, NJ, 1973.

Joy, (Admiral) C. T.; *How Communists Negotiate;* MacMillan, New York, NY, 1955.

Karrass, C. L.; *The Negotiating Game;* World, New York, NY, 1970.

Levin, L.; *Levin's Laws;* M. Evans & Co., Boston, MA, 1979.

Lieberman, M.; *Bargaining;* Teach'em, Inc., Chicago, IL, 1979.

Lockhart, C.; *Bargaining in International Conflicts;* Columbia University Press, New York, NY, 1979.

Machiavelli, N.; *The Prince;* Translated by Robert M. Adams, Norton, New York, 1977.

Neubert, C.; *How to Handle Your Own Contracts: A Layman's Guide;* Sterling Publishing Co., New York, NY, 1980.

Nierenberg, G. I.; *The Art of Negotiating;* Hawthorne Books, New York, NY, 1968.

Nierenberg, G. I. & Calero, H. H.; *Meta-Talk;* Simon & Schuster, New York, NY, 1973.

Peking's Approach to Negotiations; Selected Writings, Committee of Government Operations, US Government Printing Office, Washington, DC, 1969.

Robert, M.; *Managing Conflict from the Inside Out;* Learning Concepts, Austin, TX, 1982.

Schelling, C. C.; *The Strategy of Conflict;* Harvard University Press, Cambridge, MA, 1966.

Sexton, P.; *The New Nightingales;* Enquiry Press, New York, NY, 1982.

Schatzki, M.; *Negotiation;* Signet, NY, 1981.

Sperber, P.; *The Science of Business Negotiation;* Pilot Industries, Inc., New York, NY, 1979.

Terkel, S.; *Working;* Pantheon Books, New York, 1974.

Walton, R. E. & McKersie, R. B.; *A Behavioral Theory of Labor Negotiations;* McGraw-Hill, Inc., New York, NY, 1965.

Warschau, T. A.; *Winning by Negotiations;* McGraw-Hill, New York, NY, 1980.

Weiss, A.; *The Organization Guerrilla;* Atheneum, New York, NY, 1975.

Werther, W. B. & Lockhart, C. A.; *Labor Relations in the Health Profession;* Little-Brown & Co., Boston, MA, 1976.

Wincor, R.; *Contracts in Plain English;* McGraw-Hill, New York, NY, 1976.

Zartman, I. W. & Berman, M. R.; *The Practical Negotiator;* Yale University Press, New Haven, CT, 1982.

INDEX